CONGENITAL DIAPHRAGMATIC HERNIA – PRENATAL TO CHILDHOOD MANAGEMENT AND OUTCOMES

Edited by **Eleanor Molloy**

Congenital Diaphragmatic Hernia – Prenatal to Childhood Management and Outcomes
Edited by Eleanor Molloy

Published by InTech

Janeza Trdine 9, 51000 Rijeka, Croatia

Publishing Process Manager Bojan Rafaj

Technical Editor Teodora Smiljanic

Cover Designer InTech Design Team

Additional hard copies can be obtained from orders@intechopen.com

Congenital Diaphragmatic Hernia – Prenatal to Childhood Management and Outcomes,
Edited by Eleanor Molloy
p. cm.
ISBN 978-953-51-0670-8

For EU product safety concerns:
IN TECH d.o.o., Prolaz Marije Krucifikse Kozulić 3, 51000 Rijeka, Croatia,
info@intechopen.com or visit our website at intechopen.com.

Meet the editor

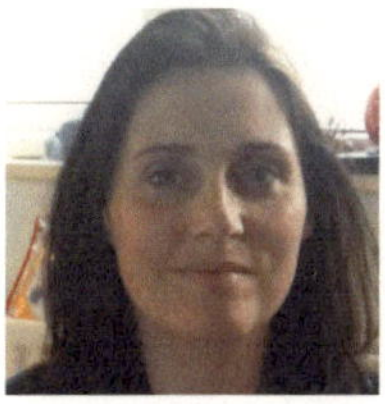

Eleanor Molloy MB, BCh, BAO, PhD, FRCPCH, FRCPI
Dr Molloy graduated from University College Cork, Ireland and subsequently trained in pediatrics and neonatology throughout Ireland and in Cleveland, USA. She is a neonatologist in Dublin and an associate professor of pediatrics in the Royal College of Surgeons in Ireland. She has published in the areas of congenital diaphragmatic hernia and also mechanisms of neonatal inflammatory diseases.

Contents

Preface

Congenital diaphragmatic hernia (CDH) remains a common malformation of the diaphragm resulting in herniation of abdominal contents into the thoracic cavity and associated pulmonary hypoplasia. Despite advances in antenatal diagnosis and neonatal intensive care, a high morbidity and mortality persist in infants with CDH. Each chapter provides an up-to-date consensus on definitions, embryology, antenatal diagnosis, genetics, associated congenital anomalies, pathophysiology and long-term outcomes. We hope that this book will appeal to pediatricians, neonatologists, pediatric surgeons, pediatric intensivists, developmental pediatricians and other healthcare professionals who are involved in the clinical management of children with CDH.

Acknowledgements:
I would like to thank Bojan Rafaj, the publishing process manager, for his patience and encouragement. In addition many thanks to all the authors who contributed their expertise and time to make their excellent contributions.

Eleanor Molloy
National Maternity Hospital & Our Lady's Hospital for Sick Children
Royal College of Surgeons of Ireland
University College Dublin,
Ireland

Section 1

Pre and Perinatal Issues in Congenital Diaphragmatic Hernia

Congenital Diaphragmatic Hernia with Emphasis on Embryology, Subtypes, and Molecular Genetics

Bahig M. Shehata[1,2] and Jenny Lin[1]
[1]*Children's Healthcare of Atlanta, Atlanta, GA*
[2]*Emory University School of Medicine, Atlanta, GA*
USA

1. Introduction

Historians, scientists, and researchers have been fascinated by the diaphragm for many centuries. Homer first described Trojan War battle wounds with reference to the diaphragm in the 9th century B.C. From 500-430 B.C., Empedocles of Agrigentum was one of the first people to study the physiology of respiration. In this early period of medical knowledge, however, the purpose of the diaphragm bewildered scientists. Hippocrates observed the diaphragm's inherent fragility and thinness that caused it to throb at any instance of unexpected joy or sorrow. Plato hypothesized that the diaphragm was not involved with respiration but rather served as a boundary between parts of the soul. It was not until Galen in the 2nd century A.D. that the actions of the diaphragm were described as upward isovolume movements during the period of rib cage expansion in respiration(Skandalakis 2004).

In the early 17th century, the first observations of congenital diaphragmatic hernia (CDH) emerged. Through these defects, the understanding of the embryological development of the diaphragm began to form. Morgagni clearly described the hiatal hernia through the foramina of Morgagni in 1761. In 1848, Bochdalek referenced the development of the pleuroperitoneal canals while describing the hernia that formed by passing through these canals. Broman proposed the first diagram of the adult diaphragm indicating its embryonic derivatives in 1905. Wells continued the study of the diaphragm along with the pleural sacs in the mid-20th century, and Adzick diagnosed 88 of 94 infants with CDH using prenatal ultrasonography in 1985(Skandalakis 2004). With the wide range of diaphragmatic defects that have been identified, the formation of the diaphragm still remains a topic of fascination today. However, in the last decade, a spectrum of genetic loci was identified as causative genes of this defect.

2.1 Embryology

2.1.1 Normal diaphragm development

Prior to diaphragm formation, the transverse septum, one of the four components that combine into the early diaphragm, begins its descent along the vertebral column. In the third week of embryonic life, the transverse septum lies at the level of the third cervical vertebra. By the end of diaphragm development in week 8, the early diaphragm descends to its ultimate position at the first lumbar segment, secondary to the rapid growth of the vertebral column. Concurrently, the phrenic nerve arises from the third to fifth cervical vertebra and follows the diaphragm down to its final location(Skandalakis 2004).

Diaphragm development begins approximately at the fourth week of intrauterine life from four embryonic structures derived from the mesoderm: the transverse septum, the pleuroperitoneal membranes, the dorsal esophageal mesentery, and the musculature of the body wall (Figure 1)(Bielinska, Jay et al. 2007; Hartnett 2008). The transverse septum, an infolding of the ventral body wall, develops into the anterior central tendon, beginning the separation of the pleuro-pericardial cavity and the peritoneal cavity(Clugston and Greer 2007; Hartnett 2008; Keijzer and Puri 2010). The incomplete separation of the body cavities results in two openings adjacent to the esophagus called the pericardio-peritoneal canals(Hartnett 2008).

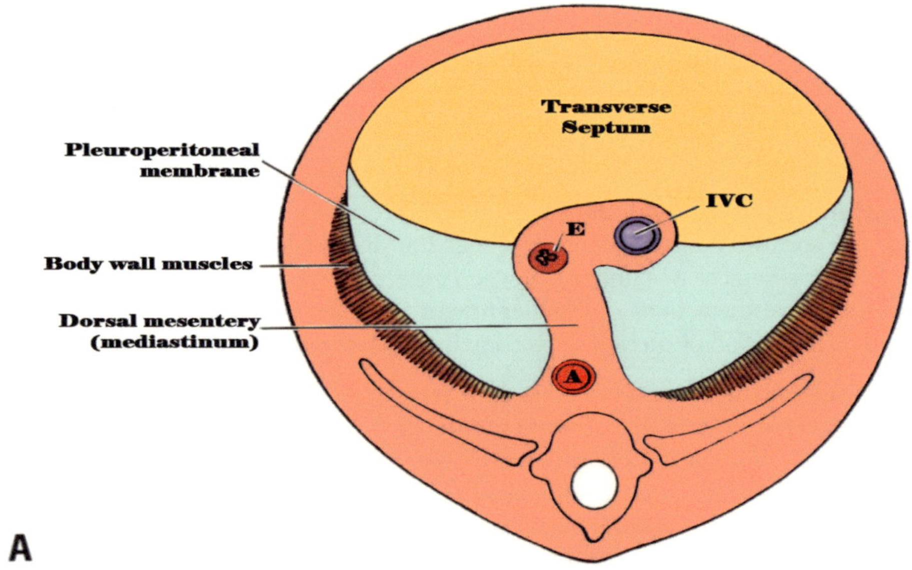

Fig. 1. Component of diaphragm, early embryonic life

Another infolding of the posterolateral body wall develops into the pleuroperitoneal membranes, which originates from the caudal end of the pericardioperitoneal canals and travels medially and ventrally(Hartnett 2008; Keijzer and Puri 2010). The fusion of the transverse septum with the pleuroperitoneal membranes and structures around the esophageal mesentery begins the closure of the pleuroperitoneal canals, with the right side closing before the left(Keijzer and Puri 2010). During weeks four to six, pleuroperitoneal folds are formed as a pair of temporary pyramidal structures joining the pleuropericardial folds to the transverse septum(Clugston and Greer 2007). Closure is completed around the eighth week of gestation (Figure 2)(Clugston and Greer 2007).

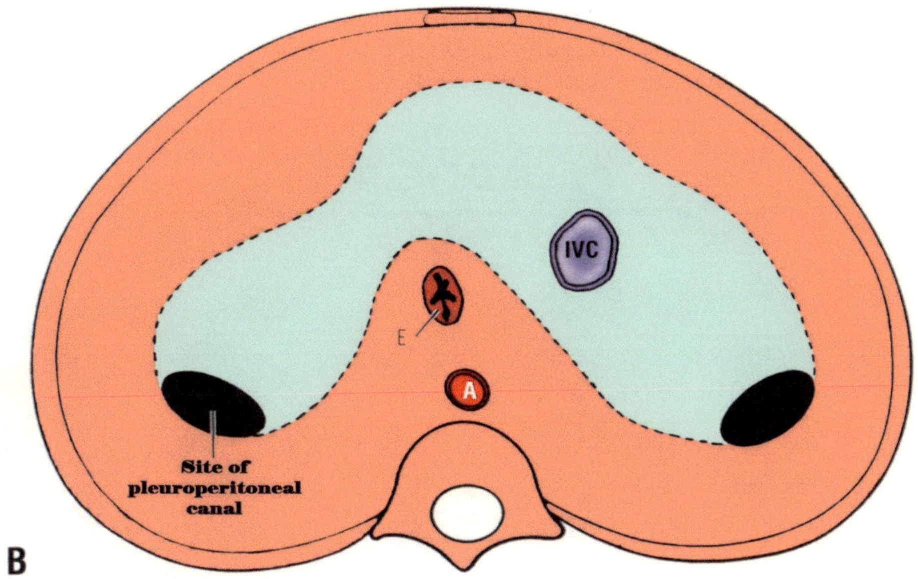

Fig. 2. Diagram showing sites of closure in normally developed diaphragm

After the early diaphragm is formed, distinct myogenic cells migrate from the lateral dermomyotomal lip and invade the pleuroperitoneal folds(Clugston and Greer 2007). The muscle precursor cells then proliferate and radiate out to muscularize the entire diaphragm(Clugston and Greer 2007). Simultaneously, the phrenic nerve extends to the pleuroperitoneal folds and, from there, innervates the remainder of the diaphragm(Clugston and Greer 2007). The muscularization and innervation of the diaphragm is concluded at about week ten(Clugston and Greer 2007).

2.2 Abnormal diaphragm development

Many theories have been proposed as to the cause of diaphragmatic hernias. In one theory, abdominal viscera herniate through the diaphragm to prevent closure. The presence of the viscera in the thoracic cavity then leads to pulmonary hypoplasia. In another theory, the primary insult is believed to be pulmonary hypoplasia. This is followed by the abdominal viscera migrating into the chest as a result of a lack of adequate pulmonary parenchyma. The diaphragm then fails to fuse due to the invading abdominal viscera. It has also been hypothesized in yet another theory that the same embryological accident produces pulmonary hypoplasia and the diaphragmatic defect. No theory is proven at this time. However, more support lends to the latter two theories from animal studies.

Diaphragmatic hernia can be classified under two major categories, congenital and acquired. The congenital diaphragmatic hernias are classified as 1) posterior lateral defect of the diaphragm (Bochdalek), 2) anterior defect of the diaphragm (Morgagni), 3) peritoneopericardial central diaphragmatic hernia (septum transverse type), 4) eventration of the diaphragm, 5) hiatal hernia and paraesophageal hernia, (6) and others(Skandalakis 2004). Of the congenital hernias, Bochdalek and Morgagni represent the majority of cases of CDH (Figure 3). On the other hand, acquired diaphragmatic hernias are traumatic in nature(Skandalakis 2004).

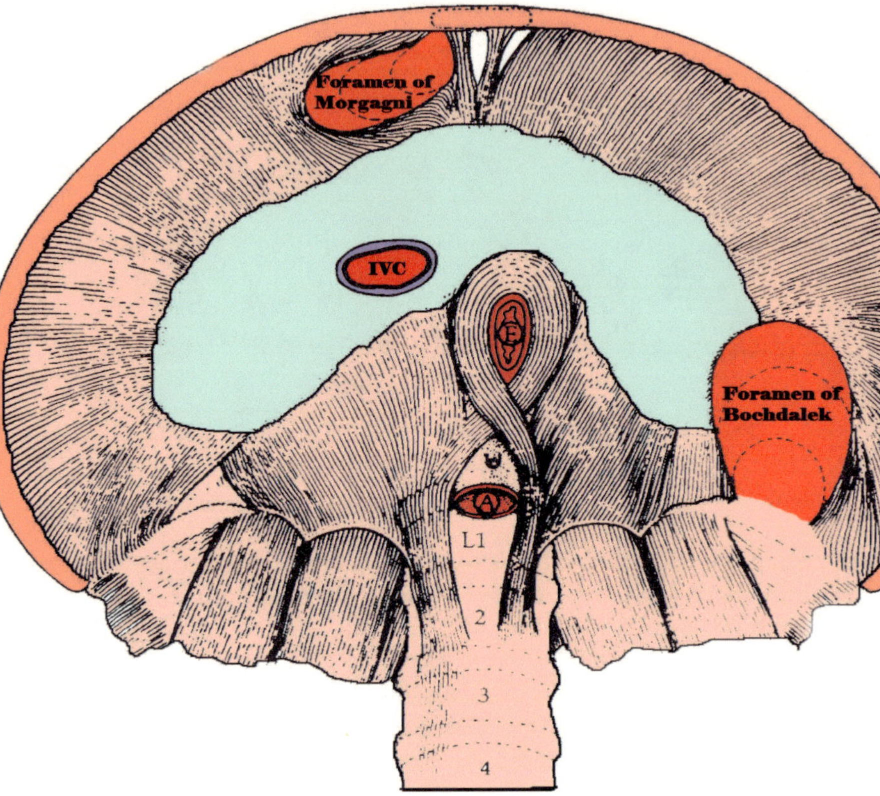

Fig. 3. Diagram showing the site of Bochdalek and Morgagni defects

2.2.1 Congenital diaphragmatic hernia

2.2.1.1 Posterior lateral defect of the diaphragm (Bochdalek)

This defect represents over 70% of diaphragmatic hernias. It begins above and lateral to the left lateral arcuate ligament at the vertebral costal trigone. The event occurs during the intestinal return to the abdominal cavity around the 10th week of embryonic life. At that time, the trigone is composed mainly of membranous tissue with rare muscle fibers. The increased intra-abdominal pressure causes the separation of the muscle fibers and creates the defect. The defect can be small in size or, in extreme cases, almost the entire hemidiaphragm is involved. Approximately 90% of this defect occurs on the left side while the right side represents less than 10% (Figure 4-5). In 99% of the cases it is unilateral. Herniation of the small intestines, stomach, colon, spleen, and part of the liver may occur (Figure 6-7)(Skandalakis 2004). Subsequently, pulmonary hypoplasia with mediastinal shift occurs.

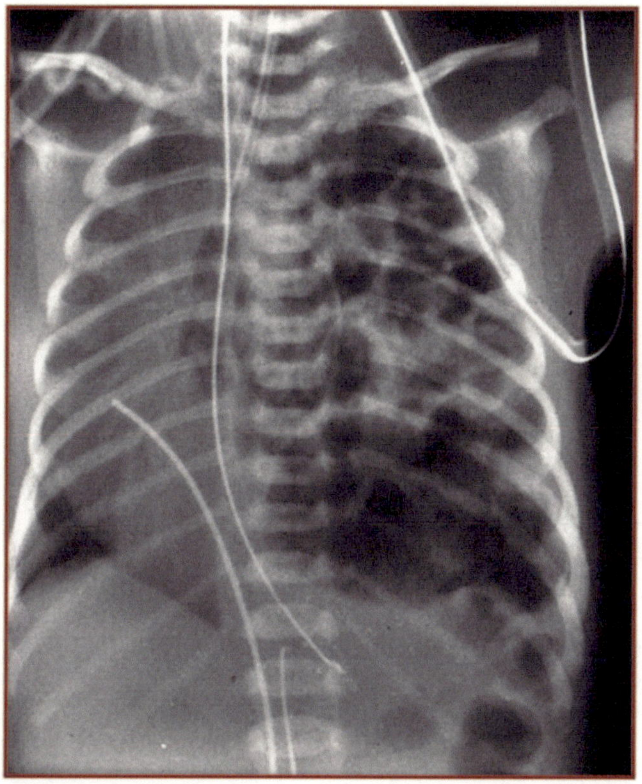

Fig. 4. X-ray of left diaphragmatic hernia

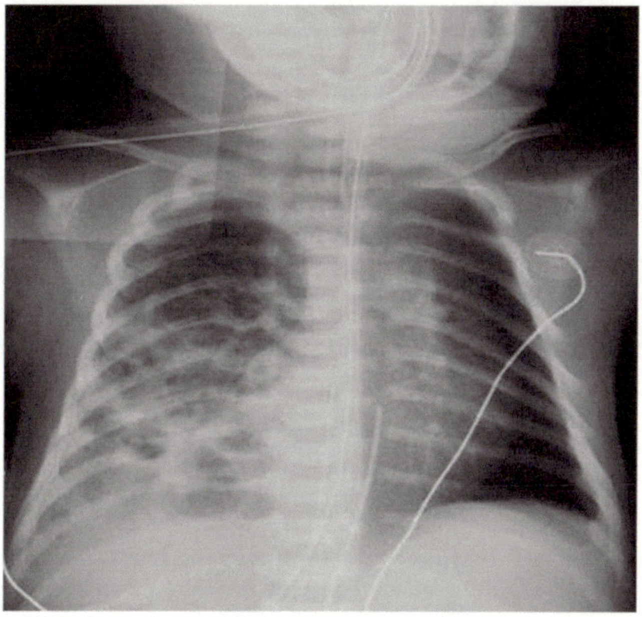

Fig. 5. X-ray of right diaphragmatic hernia

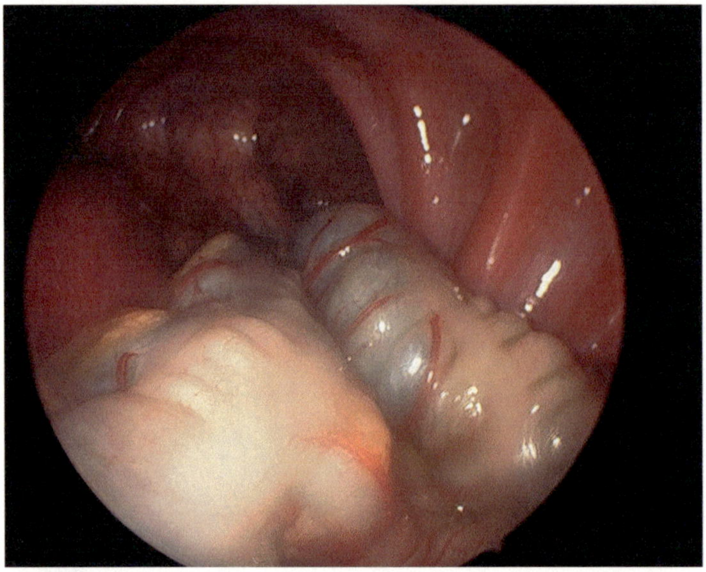

Fig. 6. Colon herniating through the Bochdalek diaphragmatic hernia

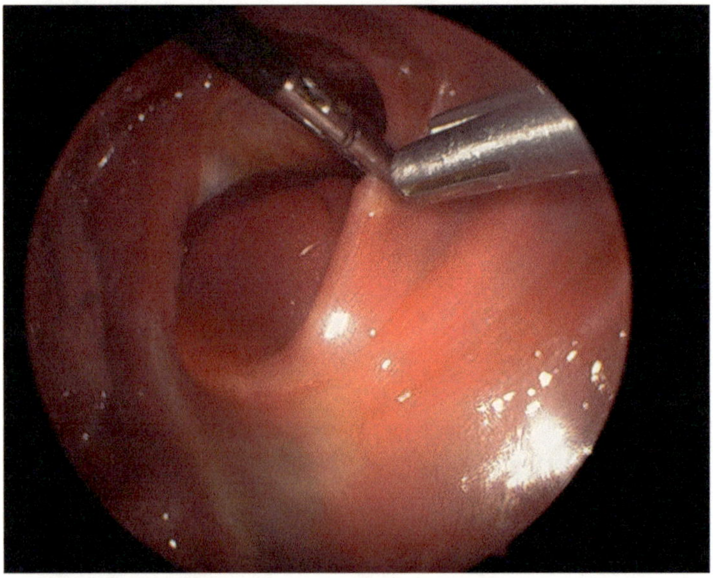

Fig. 7. Spleen herniating through the Bochdalek diaphragmatic hernia

2.2.1.2 Anterior defect of the diaphragm (Morgagni)

This is also known as parasternal defect of the diaphragm, which results from a small gap of the musculature on either side of the xiphoid process and the seventh costal cartilage(Skandalakis 2004). It occurs from a failure of the crural and sterna portions of the diaphragm to fuse. It is usually associated with omental herniation, hence they always contain fat(Gossios, Tatsis et al. 1991). 90% of the Morgagni type occurs on the right side, and 7% occur bilaterally.

2.2.1.3 Peritoneopericardial central diaphragmatic hernia (septum transverse type)

This rare type has been reported in newborn infants and even adults. It represents a defect in the central tendon and overlying pericardium. Incarceration of the intestines can be the early symptoms(Skandalakis 2004). The defect allows a rare occasion herniation of the liver into the pericardial sac(Davies, Oksenberg et al. 1993).

2.2.1.4 Eventration of the diaphragm

It can be classified into congenital or traumatic. It occurs when the entire leaf of the diaphragm bulges upward (Figure 8). It is more common on the left side and affects males more than females, and it is usually associated with intestinal malrotation. Additionally, sigmoid valvulus and rarely gastric valvulus can be seen with this type of herniation(Tsunoda, Shibusawa et al. 1992; McIntyre, Bensard et al. 1994). It occurs mainly due to the failure of muscularization of the diaphragm leaflets, not due to fusion of the embryonic components as in the previous three entities. In the congenital form, the phrenic nerve is intact, and the lung on the affected side is collapsed but not hypoplastic.

On the other hand, the acquired eventration is due to phrenic nerve injury with normal muscularization of the diaphragmatic leaflets(Skandalakis 2004).

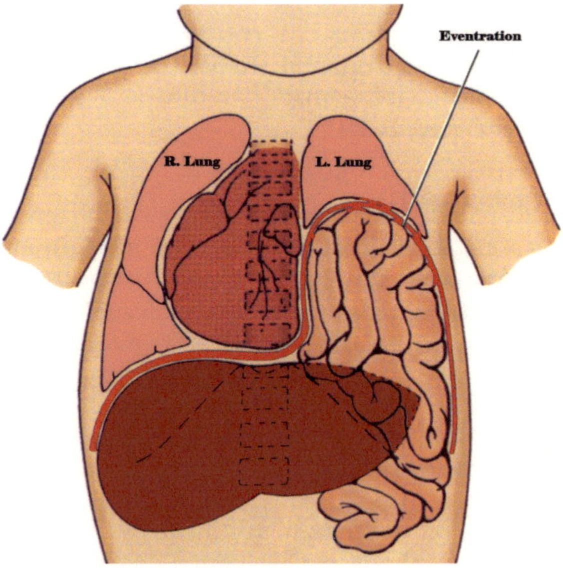

Fig. 8. Diagram showing eventration of the diaphragm

2.2.1.5 Hiatal hernia

This lesion results from an enlarged hiatus and a weakened phrenoesophageal ligament. It can be classified into two subtypes, sliding hiatal hernia and paraesophageal hernia. In the sliding hiatal hernia, a part of the stomach is placed upward with the gastroesophageal junction located in the thoracic cavity. In the paraesophageal hernia, the gastroesophageal junction is normally located below the diaphragm. However, the portion of the fundis can herniate into the thoracic cavity anterior to the esophagus, and, on rare occasions, a piece of omentum can be seen in the thoracic cavity(Skandalakis 2004).

2.2.1.6 Others

Accessory diaphragm and duplication of diaphragm

This rare anomaly divides the corresponding hemothorax into two spaces by an accessory sheet of fibromuscular tissue. The origin of the membrane usually comes from the pericardial reflection. It can be attached to the seventh rib. However, in rare occasions, it can be attached to the apex of the pleural. The lower cavity of the hemothorax usually contains a hypoplastic portion of the lung(Skandalakis 2004).

A true duplication rarely occurs secondary to the duplication of the septum transversum(Krzyzaniak and Gray 1986).

Diaphragmatic agenesis

This rare entity occurs secondary to the failure of the diaphragmatic components or their failure to join properly in the early embryonic life. It usually occurs unilaterally(Skandalakis 2004). However, in rare occasions, bilateral agenesis can occur especially in association with pentalogy of Cantrell.

2.2.2 Acquired/traumatic hernia

This entity is rare and usually results from post-natal trauma. It is more common in the right side with a portion of omentum, colon, and stomach herniated into the thoracic cavity. Another rare form represents diaphragmatic rupture and rib fracture resulting from paraoxysmal coughing(Skandalakis 2004).

2.2.3 Abnormal lung development

Although repairing a diaphragmatic defect in a newborn is relatively simple via a primary closure or a patch, the major issue is that the development of the lungs is disrupted, causing pulmonary hypoplasia and constant pulmonary hypertension(van Loenhout, Tibboel et al. 2009; Keijzer and Puri 2010). Pulmonary hypoplasia, reduced airway branching, and surfactant deficiency in newborns with CDH result in respiratory failure at birth(Keijzer and Puri 2010). Children with a CDH suffer from significant levels of morbidity and mortality due to abnormal pulmonary development. Improved treatment of newborns with CDH in the neonatal intensive care unit has substantially reduced mortality rates to less than 10% to 20% in tertiary referral centers(van Loenhout, Tibboel et al. 2009; Keijzer and Puri 2010). The high morbidity rate is attributed to modern treatment methods, such as high-frequency oscillation and extracorporeal membrane oxygenation (ECMO) (van Loenhout, Tibboel et al. 2009; Keijzer and Puri 2010).

Pulmonary hypoplasia is thought to be the result of a dual-hit hypothesis. Traditionally, it was believed that a hypoplastic lung developed only with the diaphragmatic hernia. In the dual-hit hypothesis, however, the lungs suffer from two insults, the first one inherent in pulmonary development before the development of the CDH and the second insult occurring with the CDH. The lungs are inherently disturbed prior to the early formation of the diaphragm before any mechanical pressure can be applied by the CDH(van Loenhout, Tibboel et al. 2009; Keijzer and Puri 2010). A second insult to the ipsilateral lung subsequently occurs as a result of disturbance of fetal breathing movements due to the abdominal organs invading the thoracic cavity(van Loenhout, Tibboel et al. 2009; Keijzer and Puri 2010). Although some authors have postulated that the hypoplastic lung causes the diaphragmatic hernia, animal models of mutant mice with inactivated *Fgf10*, thereby preventing lung development, still had normal diaphragms, disproving that abnormal pulmonary growth creates the diaphragmatic defect(Keijzer and Puri 2010).

2.2.4 Associated anomalies

Many anomalies have been associated with CDH, including intestinal malrotation, congenital heart defects, pulmonary stenosis, tracheal agenesis, abdominal wall defects (omphalocele and gastroschisis), obstructive uropathy, skeletal anomalies (in particular vertebral malformation), choanal atresia, and neural tube defect(Skandalakis 2004). Additionally, the instance of CDH is seen more frequently in syndromic infants, particularly with trisomy 18, trisomy 21, and pentalogy of Cantrell (Figure 9-10).

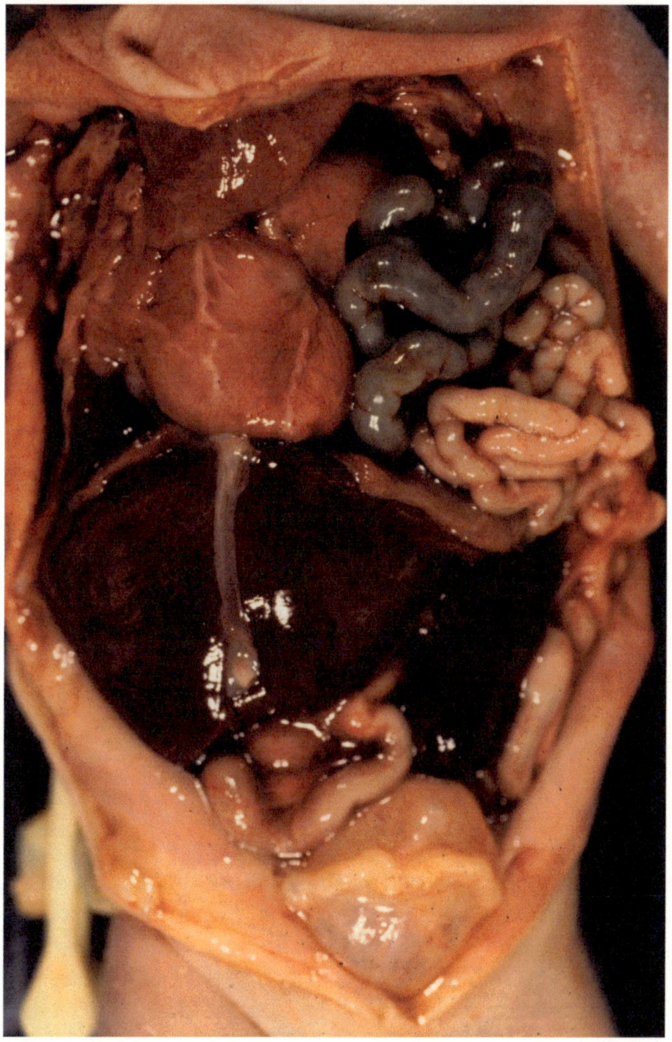

Fig. 9. Fetus with trisomy 18 and left diaphragmatic hernia

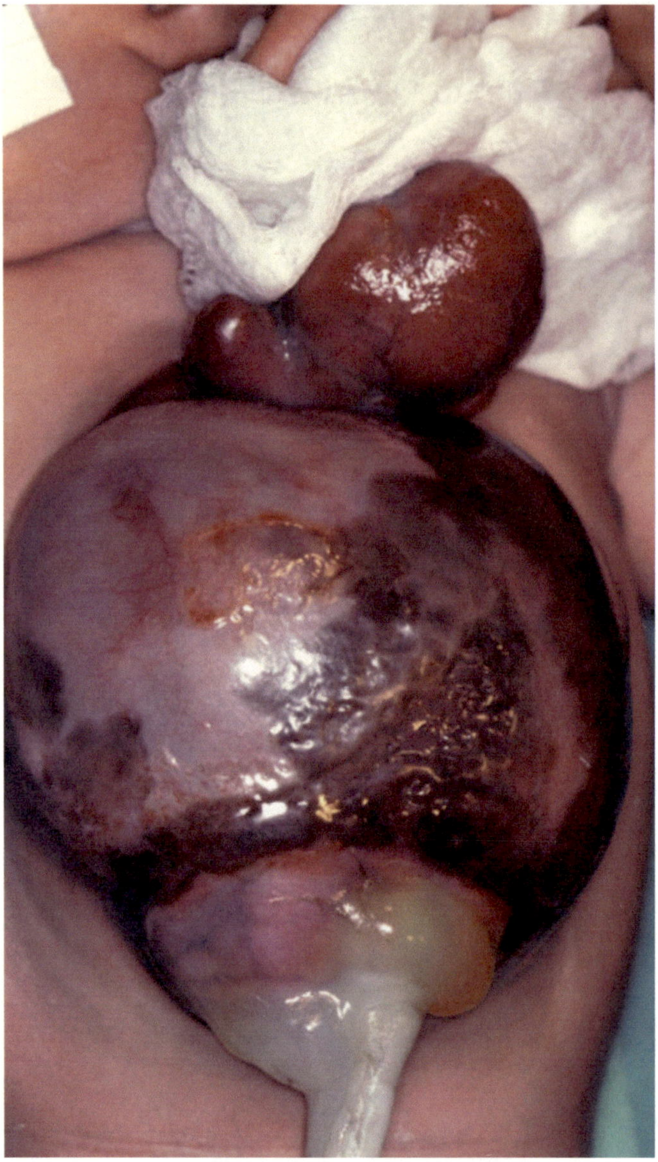

Fig. 10. Fetus with pentalogy of Cantrell and ectopia cordis

3. Molecular genetics

A genetic component has been confirmed in the etiology of CDH(Bielinska, Jay et al. 2007). However, many genes have been implicated in its pathogenesis, which may be the cause of multiple developmental insults during embryological growth of the diaphragm and lung(van Loenhout, Tibboel et al. 2009). The phenotype of CDH has been observed to be significantly variable, suggesting that its etiology is most likely due to more than one single gene mutation(van Loenhout, Tibboel et al. 2009). Moreover, it has been hypothesized that CDH may also be influenced by environmental factors, increasing the complexity in determining the specific genetic mutations that may induce diaphragmatic defects(van Loenhout, Tibboel et al. 2009).

Despite this multifactorial nature of CDH, various genes have been identified and associated in CDH. Transcriptional regulators have been hypothesized to contribute to the development of CDH(Bielinska, Jay et al. 2007). Transcription factor haploinsufficiency in humans is an accepted cause of CDH, especially when it is accompanied with other congenital defects(Bielinska, Jay et al. 2007). Transcription factors can regulate gene expression for mesenchymal cell function, and if impaired, they can cause impaired structure, apoptosis, and anomalous cell sorting(Bielinska, Jay et al. 2007).

Factors of cell migration, mesodermal patterning, or the structure of extracellular matrix have also been implicated in the morphogenesis of CDH(Bielinska, Jay et al. 2007). Mutations in genes directing cell migration and mesodermal patterning are essential for growth/guidance factors, receptors, and parts of the extracellular matrix (ECM) and have been related to CDH and extradiaphragmatic defects(Bielinska, Jay et al. 2007). The mesenchymal hit hypothesis proposes that signaling pathways common to cells in organs derived from the mesoderm are disturbed by genetic and environmental triggers in CDH(Bielinska, Jay et al. 2007). Thus, it is not surprising that diaphragmatic defects are often accompanied by abnormalities in the heart, lungs, and liver in nonisolated CDH(Bielinska, Jay et al. 2007).

In addition, the development of the diaphragm is dependent on proteins involved in the metabolism and binding of retinoids, and animal studies have shown that 25-40% of rat offspring develop a CDH when fed a vitamin A deficient diet(Goumy, Gouas et al. 2010; Keijzer and Puri 2010). In chromosome loci commonly associated with CDH, identified genes involved in the retinoic signaling pathway have been proposed as causative pathways of CDH(Goumy, Gouas et al. 2010).

3.1 Wt1

Wilms' tumor suppressor gene, *Wt1*, is a zinc finger transcription factor expressed in the amuscular diaphragm, pleural/abdominal mesothelial cells, epicardium, testicular somatic cells, and kidney(Bielinska, Jay et al. 2007). Heterozygous mutations in *Wt1* are known to cause syndromic CDH, such as Wilms' tumor-Aniridia-Genitourinary anomalies-mental Retardation (WAGR), Denys-Drash, Frasier, and Meacham syndrome(Bielinska, Jay et al. 2007; van Loenhout, Tibboel et al. 2009). Symptoms of these syndromes include genitourinary, diaphragmatic, and cardiac deformations(Bielinska, Jay et al. 2007). Although no mutations in *Wt1* have been linked to isolated CDH in humans, a Bochdalek hernia originating from the deformation of the pleuroperitoneal folds was observed in *Wt1* null mutant mice, along with cardiac abnormalities(Clugston and Greer 2007).

3.2 Fog2

Friend of GATA-2, a multi-zinc finger transcription factor that binds to the *Gata* transcription factor family, is expressed in mesodermal tissue, such as the early diaphragm, lung mesenchyme, epicardium, myocardium, and testicular somatic cells(Bielinska, Jay et al. 2007; Goumy, Gouas et al. 2010). It lies on chromosome 8q23, and a nonsense mutation in a female patient with severe bilateral pulmonary hypoplasia and a posterior diaphragmatic eventration on the left side(Bielinska, Jay et al. 2007; van Loenhout, Tibboel et al. 2009; Keijzer and Puri 2010). Rearrangements of *Fog2* in two cases of isolated CDH were found but not identified as mutations(van Loenhout, Tibboel et al. 2009). Patients with loss-of-function point mutations heterozygous for *Fog2* can develop diaphragm anomalies (eventration), pulmonary hypoplasia, and/or cardiac abnormalities(Bielinska, Jay et al. 2007). *Fog2* is the only gene thus far identified with mutations in nonsyndromic CDH patients, supporting its importance in diaphragmatic and lung development in humans.

Animal studies have displayed that a mutation in this gene causes severe pulmonary hypoplasia with a posterolateral muscularization defect instead of a developmental defect, supporting the notion that the defects of the lungs and diaphragm in CDH occur separately(van Loenhout, Tibboel et al. 2009).

3.3 Gata-4

The zinc finger transcription factor *Gata4*, which interacts with *Fog2*, is also expressed in mesenchymal cells of the embryological diaphragm, lungs, heart, and testicular somatic cells(Bielinska, Jay et al. 2007; van Loenhout, Tibboel et al. 2009). *Gata4* lies on chromosome 8p23.1 and is known to be involved in heart development(Wat, Shchelochkov et al. 2009). Patients heterozygous for *Gata4* loss-of-function mutations with terminal deletions extending to at least 8p23.1 developed cardiac deformations, and microdeletions on 8p23.1 have been linked to a spectrum of cardiac malformations, such as atrioventricular septal defects, hypoplastic left heart, hypoplastic right ventricle, pulmonary atresia/stenosis, pulmonary valve stenosis, partial anomalous pulmonary venous return, subaortic stenosis, transposition of the great arteries, double-inlet/double-outlet right ventricle, and tetralogy of Fallot(Wat, Shchelochkov et al. 2009). Haploinsufficiency of *Sox7* with Gata4 deletions may worsen these cardiac conditions(Wat, Shchelochkov et al. 2009).

Isolated CDH is also common in patients with *Gata4* deletions in at least nine previous cases(van Loenhout, Tibboel et al. 2009; Wat, Shchelochkov et al. 2009). CDH has occurred with 22.2% of patients with reported interstitial deletions of 8p23.1, and the majority of these patients have developed left-sided CDH(Wat, Shchelochkov et al. 2009).

In animal studies, 70% of mice heterozygous for *Gata4* knockout mutations developed heart, lung and midline diaphragmatic defects(van Loenhout, Tibboel et al. 2009). The midline diaphragm malformation was described as a ventral hernia covered by a sac that allowed the abdominal viscera to protrude and was present in about 30% of the mice(Bielinska, Jay et al. 2007; Wat, Shchelochkov et al. 2009). Moreover, it has been shown that *Gata4* is important for normal pulmonary lobar development(van Loenhout, Tibboel et al. 2009).

3.4 Coup-TFII

Chicken ovalbumin upstream promoter-transcription factor II (*Coup-TFII*) is a nuclear orphan receptor of *Fog2* that belongs to a steroid/thyroid hormone receptor superfamily and is expressed in a variety of tissues, including mesodermal tissues in the diaphragm, lungs, and heart(Bielinska, Jay et al. 2007; van Loenhout, Tibboel et al. 2009). The minimally deleted region on human chromosome 15q26.1-26.2 has been identified in CDH patients, and *Coup-TFII* is one of the four genes that is located in this region, suggesting its possible involvement in the CDH of patients with 15q deletions(Bielinska, Jay et al. 2007). However, in a review of over 130 cases, no mutations in *Coup-TFII* were found(van Loenhout, Tibboel et al. 2009). Mutations in this gene were also absent in 73 CDH cases tested by Scott et al. and in over 100 cases reviewed by Slavotinek et al.(Goumy, Gouas et al. 2010).

Despite the lack of evidence of *Coup-TFII* in the implication of CDH, animal studies have proven to be more convincing. Mice with Cre-lox conditional mutagenesis of *Coup-TFII* in the mesenchyme and pleuroperitoneal folds developed diaphragm malformations similar to Bochdalek diaphragmatic hernias(Bielinska, Jay et al. 2007; van Loenhout, Tibboel et al. 2009). In these studies, *Coup-TFII* expression was shown to be significantly downregulated in the early diaphragm and pleuroperitoneal folds but only slightly reduced in the early lung(van Loenhout, Tibboel et al. 2009). Upregulation of *Coup-TFII* may cause hypoplastic lung in the nitrofen rat model through a negative feedback system during diaphragm development (Goumy, Gouas et al. 2010; Keijzer and Puri 2010). *Coup-TFII* null mice show malformations in cardiovascular development(Goumy, Gouas et al. 2010; Keijzer and Puri 2010).

3.5 Shh signaling pathway

Sonic Hedgehog (*Shh*) and *Gli2* and *Gli3* are highly conserved genes that are components of the *Shh* signaling pathway(van Loenhout, Tibboel et al. 2009). *Shh* has been shown to be a vital protein for the morphogenesis of the early respiratory system in the mouse embryo(Goumy, Gouas et al. 2010). In *Shh* null mutant mice, tracheo-esophageal separation is absent, and the branching of the lungs is underdeveloped, forming hypoplastic lungs(van Loenhout, Tibboel et al. 2009). In the nitrofen rat model of CDH and in the hypoplastic lungs of CDH patients, *Shh* has been shown to be downregulated(van Loenhout, Tibboel et al. 2009; Goumy, Gouas et al. 2010).

Similarly, animal studies have shown that *Gli2* and *Gli3* mutant mice have similar foregut anomalies with a more severe lack of pulmonary branching. In the original publication on the functions of *Shh* and *Gli2* and *Gli3*, mutants of *Gli2* and *Gli3* mice demonstrated more severe failure of pulmonary branching, ranging from failure of primary branching to the agenesis of the lungs to ectopic branching and fusion of both lungs(van Loenhout, Tibboel et al. 2009). No diaphragmatic in this study was reported(van Loenhout, Tibboel et al. 2009). However, in a more recent study conducted by the same authors showed that *Gli2* and *Gli3* null mutant mice showed evidence of CDH(van Loenhout, Tibboel et al. 2009; Keijzer and Puri 2010). Evidence that *Gli2* and *Gli3* play roles in CDH in human patients has yet to be found(van Loenhout, Tibboel et al. 2009).

3.6 Slit3 and Robo1

Slit3 belongs to the *Slit* family proteins, which are secreted molecules involved in axon guidance through repulsion and mesodermal cell migration(Bielinska, Jay et al. 2007; van Loenhout, Tibboel et al. 2009). This gene is expressed in the embryonic diaphragm among other tissues(Bielinska, Jay et al. 2007). Seventy percent of null mutant mice have displayed central-type diaphragmatic hernias, cardiac defects, and renal deformations(Bielinska, Jay et al. 2007; van Loenhout, Tibboel et al. 2009). This diaphragmatic defect is derived from abnormal connective tissue formation in the central septum transversum, which causes liver attachment on the right side, creating a likeness to the human central CDH(van Loenhout, Tibboel et al. 2009). Moreover, these mice do not experience pulmonary hypoplasia and do not die of respiratory failure(Keijzer and Puri 2010). One newborn with CDH was observed to have a hernia sac attached to the liver, similar to the *Slit3* null mutant mice(van Loenhout, Tibboel et al. 2009).

Robo1 is a surface transmembrane protein and receptor of *Slit3* found in the brain, lung, heart, liver, muscle, and kidney(Bielinska, Jay et al. 2007). *Robo1*$^{-/-}$ mice die upon birth from respiratory failure and have abnormal mesenchymal cellularity, with some displaying CDH(Bielinska, Jay et al. 2007).

No mutations of *Slit3* or *Robo1* have been found in patients with CDH(Bielinska, Jay et al. 2007). However, mutations in heparan sulfate, a proteoglycan possibly essential to the signaling complex of *Slit3* and *Robo1*, have been discovered in CDH patients(Bielinska, Jay et al. 2007).

3.7 PDGFRα

Platelet-derived growth factor receptor-α (*PDGFRa*), known to be involved in the formation of gastrointestinal and neural tumors, was recently identified to be significant in the morphogenesis of the diaphragm and lung(van Loenhout, Tibboel et al. 2009). In *PDGFRα* null mice, pulmonary hypoplasia and posterolateral diaphragmatic hernias were found, similar to Fryns syndrome, a nonisolated CDH found in humans(van Loenhout, Tibboel et al. 2009; Keijzer and Puri 2010). Moreover, a genetic sequence variant of *PDGFRa* was found in one patient with nonisolated CDH(van Loenhout, Tibboel et al. 2009). Thus, *PDGFRa* is a potential candidate for syndromic CDH.

3.8 Retinoid signaling pathway

Retinoids have a major role in various biological processes, including embryogenesis and lung development(Goumy, Gouas et al. 2010). Increasing evidence in animal studies has recognized the retinoid signaling pathway as an important factor in the development of the diaphragm. For instance, 25-40% of rat offspring fed a diet deficient in vitamin A developed diaphragmatic abnormalities, and this percentage decreased upon the reintroduction of vitamin A mid-gestation(Goumy, Gouas et al. 2010). Retinoic acid receptor (RAR) double mutant mice displayed posterolateral diaphragmatic defects similar to those seen in humans (van Loenhout, Tibboel et al. 2009; Goumy, Gouas et al. 2010). In another study, RALDH2, the enzyme that converts retinal into retinoic acid, was inhibited in utero by nitrofen herbicide, which caused CDH and lung deformities in rats(Goumy, Gouas et al. 2010). Moreover, by using a pan-RAR antagonist to block RAR signaling, results showed a high level of left-sided CDH(Goumy, Gouas et al. 2010).

In humans, evidence has begun to support the role of retinoids in CDH development. Retinol and retinol-binding protein plasma levels were about 50% less in newborns with CDH than healthy newborns(Goumy, Gouas et al. 2010). Also, in a case of a pleiotrophic malformation syndrome including CDH, mutations of *Stra6*, a membrane receptor involved in cellular uptake of vitamin A, were found(Goumy, Gouas et al. 2010). These results support the hypothesis of the involvement of the retinoid signaling pathway in the etiology of CDH.

Many of the genes we have discussed are involved in the retinoid signaling pathway, especially genes in chromosome loci known to be associated with CDH. In chromosome 1, deletions in the 1q41-1q42 region increases the likelihood of CDH malformation(Goumy, Gouas et al. 2010). *Disp1* is a gene in this region that interacts in the *Shh* pathway, which targets *Coup-TFII*, a repressor of the retinoid pathway(van Loenhout, Tibboel et al. 2009; Goumy, Gouas et al. 2010). Thus, it may be possible that a loss of the *Disp1* gene may disrupt the *Shh* pathway and *Coup-TFII*, disturbing retinoic acid signaling and leading to CDH(Goumy, Gouas et al. 2010).

Chromosome 8 is frequently involved in CDH mutations. Microdeletions on chromosome 8p23.1 are common in CDH patients, where the human *Gata4* gene resides(Goumy, Gouas et al. 2010). The expression and activity of *Gata4* is modulated by retinoids and may affect its function in mesodermal embryogenesis(Goumy, Gouas et al. 2010). 8q23.1, a region found to contain deletions in 6 cases, includes the *Fog2* gene on its proximal end nearest 8q22.3(Goumy, Gouas et al. 2010). *Fog2* is indirectly involved in the retinoic acid pathway in various ways. It regulates target genes of *Gata* proteins through a heterodimer formation of the *Gata* family(Goumy, Gouas et al. 2010). *Fog2* is also a corepressor protein for *Coup-TFII* and *Gata4*, and it has been suggested that simultaneous activity of *Fog2* and *Gata4* is necessary in order to direct mesenchymal cell function(Goumy, Gouas et al. 2010).

Chromosome 15 is another chromosome that has been known to have multiple deletions in CDH cases. Four patients were described with 15q24 microdeletions along with diaphragmatic hernias(Goumy, Gouas et al. 2010). *Stra6*, mentioned previously, encodes a receptor for RBP4-retinol on cell membranes and influences cell uptake of retinol molecules(Goumy, Gouas et al. 2010). *Stra6* transcription is directly affected by retinoic acid levels(Goumy, Gouas et al. 2010). It is found to be expressed in the respiratory mesenchyme and respiratory/bronchial epithelium and is associated with severe malformations in humans, including diaphragmatic defects(Goumy, Gouas et al. 2010). 15q24 is another location on chromosome 15 that is involved in retinoic acid signaling and may be implicated in CDH etiology. Cellular retinoic acid binding protein 1 (*CRABP1*) is located in this region and encodes a lipid-binding protein that regulates intracellular concentration of retinoic acid by retinoic acid catabolism and transport from the cytoplasm to nuclear receptors(Goumy, Gouas et al. 2010).

The *Coup-TFII* gene is located on 15q26.1-q26.2 on chromosome 15, and deleted regions have been found in patients with syndromic CDH(Goumy, Gouas et al. 2010). *Coup-TFII* can regulate gene transcription and repress the retinoid pathway by preventing RAR heterodimer formation(Goumy, Gouas et al. 2010). *Fog2*, as mentioned before, is also known to interact with *Coup-TFII*, another gene involved in retinoid activity.

In chromosome 3, deletions have been found in 3 patients in literature in 3q21-23(Goumy, Gouas et al. 2010). Retinol-binding protein 1 and 2 (*RBP1* and *RBP2*) are located at the distal end of the 3q23 band adjacent to 3q22 and encode cellular *RBP*s (*CRBPs*) involved in intracellular retinol movement(Goumy, Gouas et al. 2010).

CDH has also been diagnosed in 4 cases with deletions and duplications in chromosome 4q32.1(Goumy, Gouas et al. 2010). The *LRAT* gene is located in this region, and it translates into a microsomal enzyme that catalyzes the esterification of retinol for retinoid homeostasis(Goumy, Gouas et al. 2010). A downregulation of *LRAT* found in nitrofen models caused a shift of retinol homeostasis, disrupting the balance of the converted and stored forms(Goumy, Gouas et al. 2010). This suggested that nitrofen blocks retinoid pathways earlier than *RALDH*, the protein previously thought to be inhibited by nitrofen(Goumy, Gouas et al.

2010). Other molecules involved in the retinoic acid pathway also interact with *LRAT*, including RARs and *Gata* transcription factors(Goumy, Gouas et al. 2010).

4. References

Bielinska, M., P. Y. Jay, et al. (2007). "Molecular genetics of congenital diaphragmatic defects." Annals Of Medicine 39(4): 261-274.

Clugston, R. D. and J. J. Greer (2007). "Diaphragm development and congenital diaphragmatic hernia." Semin Pediatr Surg 16(2): 94-100.

Davies, M., T. Oksenberg, et al. (1993). "Massive foetal pericardiomegaly causing pulmonary hypoplasia, associated with intra-pericardial herniation of the liver." Eur J Pediatr Surg 3(6): 343-347.

Gossios, K., C. Tatsis, et al. (1991). "Omental herniation through the foramen of Morgagni: diagnosis with chest computed tomography." Chest 100: 1469.

Goumy, C., L. Gouas, et al. (2010). "Retinoid pathway and congenital diaphragmatic hernia: hypothesis from the analysis of chromosomal abnormalities." Fetal Diagn Ther 28(3): 129-139.

Hartnett, K. S. (2008). "Congenital diaphragmatic hernia: advanced physiology and care concepts." Adv Neonatal Care 8(2): 107-115.

Keijzer, R. and P. Puri (2010). "Congenital diaphragmatic hernia." Semin Pediatr Surg 19(3): 180-185.

Krzyzaniak, R. and S. Gray (1986). "Accessory septum transversum: the first case report." Am Surg 52: 278.

McIntyre, R. J., D. Bensard, et al. (1994). "The pediatric diaphragm in acute gastric volvulus." J Am Coll Surg 178: 234.

Skandalakis, J. (2004). Diaphragm. Surgical Anatomy: The Embryologic and Anatomic Basis of Modern Surgery. J. Skandalakis. Athens, Greece, Paschalidis Medical Publications, Ltd. 1: 353-392.

Tsunoda, A., M. Shibusawa, et al. (1992). "Volvulus of the sigmoid colon associated with eventration of the diaphragm." Am J Gastroenterol 87: 1682.

van Loenhout, R. B., D. Tibboel, et al. (2009). "Congenital diaphragmatic hernia: comparison of animal models and relevance to the human situation." Neonatology 96(3): 137-149.

Wat, M. J., O. A. Shchelochkov, et al. (2009). "Chromosome 8p23.1 deletions as a cause of complex congenital heart defects and diaphragmatic hernia." Am J Med Genet A 149A(8): 1661-1677.

2

Diaphragmatic Paralysis - Symptoms, Evaluation, Therapy and Outcome

Issahar Ben-Dov
The Pulmonary Institute,
C. Sheba Medical Center,
Tel-Aviv University,
Sackler Medical School
Israel

1. Introduction

The diaphragm has a major role in inspiration. The muscle separates the mostly negative pressure chest cavity, from the positive pressure abdomen. The displacement of the muscle with inspiration expands the chest, augmenting the negative pleural pressure, thereby forcing air flow into the lung. However paralysis of the muscle, unilaterally or even bilaterally, is compatible with life in most cases due to effective adaptation of the other muscles of respiration. Patients with diaphragmatic paralysis may experience a wide range of symptoms: from being asymptomatic, symptomatic only with exercise, or respiratory insufficiency and death. Symptoms depends on the pre existing cardiorespiratory status, the extent of paralysis, unilateral or bilateral and on the nature of the paralysis, acute or chronic. Some symptoms are distinct and should always raise the diagnosis of diaphragmatic paralysis. The wide range of symptoms will be described, as well as the anatomical and physiological aspects in the normal and in the disease state, etiologies, work up and therapy. Unilateral and bilateral paralysis will be discussed together, despite differences in the prevalence, causes and course.

2.1 Structure and function of the normal diaphragm

The diaphragm, the most important contributor to inspiration, is one confluent uninterrupted structure, composed of a central tendon, surrounded by muscle fibers. The structure is relatively symmetric and each hemidiaphragm is innervated by the ipsilateral phrenic nerve. The muscle fibers are inserted to the sternum, lower ribs and the arcuate ligaments (Roussos & Macklem, 1982; Fell, 1998).

Due to this orientation, contraction of the fibers leads not only to a piston shape caudal displacement of the muscle, but also to elevation and expansion of the rib cage, expanding the chest cavity caudally and circumferentially, thereby forcing airflow into the lungs.

2.2 Diaphragmatic innervations and anatomy of the phrenic nerve

Each side of the diaphragm is innervated by contralateral upper motor neurons, but in some subjects it has bilateral cortical contribution. Therefore, in unilateral hemispheric stroke, muscle function is often partially preserved.

The phrenic nerve originates in the neck from cervical, $C_{3\text{-}5}$ roots, than takes a tortuous course, penetrates the posterior chest, behind the Sternomastoid muscle, between the subclavian vessels. The left phrenic nerve runs close to the thoracic duct, crossing the internal mammary arteries anteriorly, in front of the aortic arch and main pulmonary artery, approaching the anterior aspect of the pericardium between the mediastinal pleura and the pericardium. The right phrenic nerve follows the superior vena cava and the right side of the pericardium and pierces the diaphragm lateral to the vena cava hiatus and the left nerve pierces lateral to the left heart border. Each nerve divides on the surface of the diaphragm into 4 branches. After branching, the trunks penetrate and spread along the abdominal side of the muscle. The right phrenic nerve is shorter and less tortuous. Therefore, the nerves can be interrupted or damage along this long course, within the neck, chest and even abdomen (Roussos & Macklem, 1982; Fell, 1998). Due to this unique anatomy, low cervical (below C_5) processes spare the phrenic nerves and the diaphragmatic function is preserved, despite paralysis of the intercostals muscles.

3.1 Physiology of breathing in diaphragmatic paralysis

When paralyzed, caudal displacement of the muscle with contraction is abolished or diminished, limiting chest expansion. Furthermore, due to more negative pleural pressure with inspiration, the muscle is displaced cephalad, further compromising lung inflation. The forced displacement of the diaphragm compresses the adjacent lung, thereby limiting regional ventilation. The more negative pressure that is maintained in the contralateral hemithorax causes wasted airflow from the affected to the unaffected lung. The reduced regional ventilation is often associated with reduced perfusion, but matching is not always optimal and relatively lower ventilation leads to deranged gas exchange and resting hypoxemia.

In the supine position, and in other postures when abdominal pressure rises, such as while bending forwards, the weight of the abdominal viscera or the pressure generated in the abdomen enhance cephalad displacement of the muscle, thereby further limiting lung expansion, causing dyspnea and aggravating hypoxemia (Gibson, 1989).

3.2 Causes of diaphragmatic paralysis and diaphragmatic weakness with emphasize on unique or rare causes

Diaphragmatic paralysis is in many, up to 2/3 of the cases, idiopathic. Common causes for unilateral as for bilateral paralysis are neurologic, such as peripheral phrenic nerve injuries, motor neuron disease, neuropathies and myopathies (including metabolic and endocrine) and to some extent hemispheric stroke (Gibson, GJ; Maish, 2010). In rare situations, diaphragmatic paralysis is the presenting or the predominant symptom of motor neuron disease or myopathy. Infection (viral), tumors, trauma, or inflammation can damage the nerve throughout the long course. Even subdiaphragmatic processes and operations may damage the nerve along the branches.

Among the unique etiologies for diaphragmatic paralysis that should be considered are systemic lupus erythematosus (rarely presented with diaphragmatic weakness), neck trauma or chiropractic manipulation, central vein cannulation, occult thoracic malignancy and adverse event following bronchial arteries embolization. A relatively common cause is nerve damage, thermal, vascular or direct interruption during heart or mediastinal surgery. These postsurgical patients are often difficult to wean and the diagnosis can and should be made immediately. Diaphragmatic paralysis is also common following liver transplantation. In general, unilateral or bilateral disease share similar causes, but bilateral disease is more common in systemic processes such as myopathies or metabolic diseases.

4.1 Symptoms of diaphragmatic paralysis

Loss of part or all diaphragmatic contribution to breathing has predictable effects that cause a wide range of symptoms. The symptoms depend on several factors including: the stage of the paralysis, acute or chronic, on severity; whether the paralysis is unilateral or bilateral and on the presence (and severity) or absence of pre existing lung disease. Diaphragmatic paralysis is associated with reduced vital capacity at rest, more in the supine position. The accessory muscles of ventilation face greater load and gas exchange is deranged due to poor matching of ventilation to perfusion in the affected areas, leading to hypoxemia, at rest, and more so during sleep and exercise.

Therefore, subjects may be asymptomatic, complain of dyspnea only with effort, or complain of specific symptoms, such as orthopnea (its onset is immediate after regaining the recumbent position, in contrast with the delayed orthopnea of left heart failure), dyspnea with bending, immersion or carrying even light objects. Abdominal pain due to excessive load on the abdominal muscle was the presenting symptoms of bilateral diaphragmatic paralysis (Molho et al., 1987). Abnormal gas exchange is most important if lung disease preexists. These patients may develop respiratory insufficiency, severe hypoxia and CO_2 retention. Night sweats and other symptoms have also been reported (Ben-Dov et al, 2008) .

In acute onset paralysis, patient may feel acute distress, severe orthopnea, shoulder pain and fatigue, but symptoms usually diminish, due to either desensitization, adaptation of accessory muscles of respiration or due to full or partial recovery of the phrenic nerve itself. Therefore, diaphragmatic paralysis may imitate various cardiovascular diseases (Ben-Dov et al, 2008) and symptom are often unrecognized or attributed to pre existing lung disease (i.e., COPD), thereby avoiding further evaluation, or attributed to other organ disease (i.e., CHF), thereby subjecting the patients to unnecessary evaluation.

4.2 Acute diaphragmatic paralysis

The symptoms in acute disease are more severe. Patients describe acute onset of dyspnea and orthopnea. In the post surgical and post trauma cases, weaning from mechanical ventilation may be difficult and the symptoms are often attributed to the surgery or trauma. Patients with acute onset idiopathic paralysis may be subject to extensive work up until diagnosis is appreciated. An acute syndrome has been described, neuralgic amyotrophy (not rare among idiopathic isolated phrenic nerve neuropathy), in which following a viral disease or surgery, patients feel abrupt onset of shoulder and neck pain, preceding dyspnea and orthopnea, the outcome of unilateral or bilateral phrenic nerve neuropathy. The paralysis persists in most patients but in some it resolves or relapses (Tsao et al., 2000).

Since a viral prodrome is not rare in acute onset disease, some authors attempted antiviral therapy with Valacyclovir with some positive responses. These authors consider isolated diaphragmatic paralysis as a "Bells palsy" of the phrenic nerve (Crausman et al., 2009).

4.3 Diaphragmatic paralysis in neonates

Birth injury, nerve damage during cardiothoracic surgery or cannulation of central veins and rarely neuromuscular diseases may case unilateral and rarely bilateral paralysis (Sivan & Galvis, 1990; Simansky et al., 2002).

Diagnosis is often made only after failure to wean following surgery. Symptoms may be severe, but most are not specific, beside paradoxical movement of the abdomen. Diaphragmatic paralysis should be considered in any respiratory distress under these circumstances. Echocardiography with demonstration poor or paradoxical movement of the affected hemidiaphragm, while the infant breaths spontaneously, is considered the preferred method for diagnosis. Other methods are rarely used.

Fortunately, many infants with birth trauma associated paralysis recover spontaneously within 6-12 months, with or without restoration of diaphragmatic function. Electromyography (EMG) signals and phrenic nerve conduction following nerve stimulation provide prognostic information. If supportive care is not sufficient and mechanical ventilation is prolonged, diaphragmatic plication may lead to rapid improvement. Some authors believe that plication, in the post trauma cases is in general more effective in neonate than in adults (Simansky et al., 2002).

5.1 Diagnosis of diaphragmatic paralysis

An algorithm has been suggested for the diagnosis of diaphragmatic paralysis (Polkey et al., 1995). It is based on history, physical examination with emphasis on the presence or absence of paradoxical movement of the abdominal wall (posterior, instead of anterior displacement of the abdominal wall with inspiration). This sign is important and easily recognizable if the patient lays supine and relaxed. Paradoxical movement of the abdominal wall is almost always seen with bilateral paralysis, but common even with unilateral disease. Occasionally, no paradoxical movement of the abdominal wall, but limited or asymmetrical excursion of the affected side abdominal wall can be seen. However, paradoxical movement of the abdominal wall is occasionally present in healthy subjects, especially if not relaxed during the examination.

5.2 Imaging

Diaphragmatic paralysis is usually suspected when asymmetric diaphragmatic elevation is seen on plane chest radiograph. This finding is commonly associated with linear shadows or patchy atelectasis above the paralyzed diaphragm. Asymmetric level is absent in bilateral paralysis, rendering recognition more difficult. When suspected, diaphragmatic paralysis should be confirmed by the highly sensitive sniff test, using fluoroscopy or ultrasound (Tarver et al., 1989; Gotesman & McCool, 1997). During the sniff manoeuvre, the paradoxical movement of the paralyzed hemidiaphragm, cephalad with inspiration, in contrast with the rapid caudal movement of the unaffected muscle, can be seen with fluoroscopy, while failure of the thin muscle to thicken with contraction can be seen with ultrasonography.

5.3 Lung function

With unilateral diaphragmatic paralysis, lung function usually reveals mild restriction. Baseline upright vital capacity is mildly reduced (up to 80% of predicted). With bilateral disease, vital capacity may fall to 50% of predicted (Mier-Jedrzejowicz et al., 1988). Maximal inspiratory pressures fall to 80 and 30% of predict, with unilateral and bilateral paralysis, respectively (Steier et al., 2007). Vital capacity and oxygen saturation fall is augmented in the supine position; vital capacity is at least 10% lower than in the upright position. This postural effect is larger in right side and in bilateral paralysis. The larger effect of right paralysis is probably due to the right lung being larger and due to the weight of the liver, that in the supine position promotes cephalad displacement of the muscle. Oxygen saturation often falls markedly during sleep, mainly during the REM phase, as with exercise. Diffusion capacity may be near normal in diaphragmatic paralysis and if markedly abnormal, it justifies a search for an alternative cause.

5.4.1 Additional studies

The studies described above are usually sufficient to establish the diagnosis of diaphragmatic paralysis or of severe diaphragmatic dysfunction. However, in some cases more specific measures are needed.

5.4.2 Trans diaphragmatic pressure

During inspiration, pleural pressure, reflected by esophageal pressure, becomes more negative while the pressure in the abdomen, measured via a gastric balloon, becomes more positive (abdominal content is compressed by the descending diaphragm). In contrast, with paralysis, especially when bilateral, the diaphragms are displaced cephalad due to the negative pleural pressure, so that abdominal pressure decreases instead of increasing. Therefore, normally with inspiration, esophageal pressure (negative) and the gastric pressure (positive) will change to opposite directions. In contrast, with bilateral diaphragmatic paralysis, the pressure tracing in both organs will move to the negative direction and this is the gold standard finding to document paralysis. Transdiaphragmatic pressure can be measured during spontaneous tidal, maximal or sniff manoeuvre and or following electrical phrenic nerve stimulation (using surface neck electrodes). These measurements however are difficult to standardize in bilateral disease and even more so with unilateral disease (Laporta & Grassino, 1985; American Thoracic Society/European Respiratory Society, 2002).

5.4.3 EMG

The EMG response of the diaphragm can be measured at the muscle insertion intercostals spaces with surface electrodes, with or without electrical phrenic nerve stimulation. Signals and nerve conduction velocity are studied for patterns indicating neuropathy, myopathy or show evidence of complete nerve interruption. However, these studies need expertise and are rarely performed, unless as a prerequisite for pacing.

6.1 Recommended further work up when the diagnosis of diaphragmatic paralysis is established

When diaphragmatic paralysis is confirmed, there is need to find the causal mechanism. There are no systematic studies assessing the yield of work up algorithms in an attempt to find the cause in the individual patient. However, even though most cases are idiopathic, in up to 5%, thoracic malignancy is present. Therefore, when the cause is not obvious, we recommend imaging studies, including CT scanning. Diaphragmatic paralysis, at all age groups, may be an early expression of systemic diseases, such as SLE, metabolic or endocrine disease and or of motor neuron disease, all of which justify specific evaluation, such as thyroid function and muscle enzymes and these diseases should be treated when possible.

Sleep study should be considered, since disturbed sleep is a predictable consequence of diaphragmatic paralysis (Qureshi, 2009).

7.1 Differential diagnosis

Diaphragmatic elevation, dyspnea and orthopnea may result from many other causes. It is usually easy to differentiate subpulmonic effusion or subdiaphragmatic processes by appropriate imaging. Eventration of the diaphragm, mostly congenital, is a localized fibrous replacement of part of the musculature and the lateral chest x ray shows the localized nature of the defect. Patient with other diseases may experience symptoms mimicking to those induced by diaphragmatic paralysis. Orthopnea of cardiac origin has slow onset, while that of diaphragmatic paralysis is more abrupt and is relived immediately after resuming the upright position.

8.1 Treatment options

Most patients with unilateral diaphragmatic paralysis need no specific therapy. Symptomatic patients or those with preexisting lung disease, or bilateral disease, especially if marked orthopnea exists, may benefit from non invasive nocturnal ventilatory support and this mode of therapy may offer improvement in sleep quality, day function and arterial blood gases. The rationale for anti viral therapy for patient with acute onset disease following a "viral" prodrome has been discussed earlier.

8.2 Diaphragmatic plication

The loose, paralyzed diaphragm can be folded and sutured so that the compliance decreases following plication. The argument in favor of plication is that the less compliant stretched muscle limits the cephalad displacement with inspiration. The lung region adjacent to the paralyzed muscle is therefore not or less compressed and regional ventilation improves. Furthermore, airflow from the affected lung to the normal lung minimizes, leading to improved ventilatory efficiency. Plication can be offered to selected, symptomatic patients, whose symptoms affect their life style (Simansky et al., 2002). The exact indications have not been established. Following plication in selected patients, with 5 years follow up, lung function, upright and supine, have been shown to improve, sitting and supine Vital Capacity was 9% and 19%, or more, higher, respectively and the supine fall of FVC after plication was only 9% while it was 32% prior to surgery. Daily activities and dyspnea have also been improved (Versteege et al., 2007; Freeman et al., 2009). However, this degree of improvement has not been consistently found (Higgs et al., 2002). Data on the effect of diaphragmatic plication on exercise tolerance, on peak exercise and on exercise gas exchange are anecdotal, in the adult as in the pediatric population.

8.3 Diaphragmatic pacing

Permanent phrenic nerve pacing is possible only if the phrenic nerve is fully intact and the muscle is functioning and even the deconditioned muscle fibers needs programmed gradual reconditioning. Ventilator dependent high cervical quadriplegics are candidates (Elefteriades et al., 1992). Pacing is rarely used in isolated, unilateral or bilateral diaphragmatic paralysis. There are inherent difficulties with pacing, such synchronization or lack of, with intercostal muscle.

9. Course and prognosis

Chronic unilateral diaphragmatic paralysis is usually asymptomatic or mildly symptomatic and the long term prognosis in the idiopathic and post traumatic cases is usually favorable. Even in the more symptomatic cases, symptoms gradually improve, either due to adaptation of the accessory muscles to the extra load of inspiration, or due to spontaneous recovery or improvement of the diaphragmatic function. Improvement has been described during follow up of months to years in various clinical settings (Gayan-Ramirez et al., 2008) and some authors believe that with time the compliance of the paralyzed muscle decreases, thereby limiting the cephalad displacement with inspiration (autoplication).

Bilateral disease carries worse prognosis, either because it is usually an expression of more severe disease and due to the marked impact of bilateral disease on respiratory mechanics. However, even patients with bilateral disease often improve, loss the dependency on ventilatory support, can live reasonable life and carry pregnancy and delivery. In some, adaptation is a result of one or more of the above mechanisms.

10. Conclusion

Diaphragmatic paralysis is a relatively common disease. In many cases it is mildly or not symptomatic. In many, the cause is idiopathic. Therefore, it is often undiagnosed or underappreciated. However, in some situations diaphragmatic paralysis causes severe, often unique symptoms (such as orthopnea and dyspnea with bending or immersion) that must direct to the appropriate work up. Diagnosis in most cases should be confirmed by the Sniff test with additional supportive tests such as upright and supine lung function and respiratory muscle forces. These tests are important for follow up. Correct diagnosis prevents unnecessary work up and facilitates recognition of various diseases (such as mediastinal tumors) some of them are treatable (such as inflamatory or endocrine diseases) and enhances work up for comorbidities, such as sleep abnormalities. In many patients no specific therapy is needed and in up to a quarter, paralysis or symptoms will improve spontaneously. The other may need nocturnal ventilatory assist. In selected cases diaphragmatic plication or pacing should be considered.

11. References

American Thoracic Society/European Respiratory Society. (2002) ATS/ERS Statement on Respiratory Muscle Testing. *Am J Respir Crit Care Med* 2002, Vol.166: pp. 520-624, ISSN 1073-449X

Ben-Dov, I., Kaminski, N., Reichert, N. Rosenman, J, & Shulimzon, T.(2008). Diaphragmatic Paralysis: a Clinical Imitator of Cardiorespiratory Diseases. *Israel Medical Association Journal*, Vol.10 (8-9), (August-September 2008): pp. 579-83. ISSN 1565-1088

Crausman, R. S., Summerhill, E. M., & McCool, F. D. (2009). Idiopathic Diaphragmatic Paralysis: Bell's Palsy of the Diaphragm? *Lung*, Vol.187(3), (May-June 2009): pp. 153-7, ISSN 1432-1750

Elfteriades, J. A., Hogan J. F., Handler, A., & Loke, J. S. (1992). Long-term Follow-up of Bilateral Pacing of the Diaphragm in Quadriplegia (letter*). N Engl J Med*, Vol. 326(21), (May 1992): pp. 1433-4, ISSN 0028-4793

Fell, S. C. (1998). The Respiratory Muscles. *Chest Surgery Clinics of North America,* Vol.8, No.2, (May 1998): pp. 281-94, ISSN 1052-3359

Gayan-Ramirez, G., Gosselin, N., Troosters, T., Bruyninckx, F., Gosselink, R., & Decramer, M. (2008). Functional Recovery of Diaphragm Paralysis: a Long-term Follow-up Study. *Respiratory Medicine*,Vol.102 (5), (May 2008): pp. 690-8, ISSN 0954-6111

Gibson, G. J. (1989). Diaphragmatic paresis: Pathophysiology, Clinical Features, and Investigation. *Thorax*, Vol.44 (11), (November 1989): pp. 960-70, ISSN 0040-6376

Gottesman, E., & McCool, F. D.; (1997). Ultrasound Evaluation of the Paralyzed Diaphragm. *Am J Respir Crit Care Med*,Vol. 155(5), (May 1997): pp. 1570-4, ISSN 1073-449X

Higgs, S. M., Hussain, A., Jackson, M. Donnelly, R. J., & Berrisford, R. G.; (2002). *Long* term Results of Diaphragm Plication for Unilateral Diaphragm Paralysis. *Eur J Cardiothorac Surg*, Vol.21 (2), (February 2002): pp. 294-7, ISSN 1010-7940

Laporta, D., & Grassino, A. (1985). Assessment of Transdiaphragmatic Pressure in Humans. *Journal of Applied Physiology*, Vol. 58 (5), (May 1985): pp. 1469-76, ISSN 8750-7587

Long-Term Follow-Up of the Functional and Physiologic results of Diaphragmatic Plication in Adults With Unilateral Diaphragmatic Paralysis. Ann Thorac Surgery, Vol.88 (4), (October 2009): pp1112-7, ISSN 0003-4975

Maish, M. S. (2010). *The Diaphragm*. Surgical Clinics of North America, Vol. 90 (5), (0ctober 2010): pp. 955-68, ISSN 1558-3171

Mier-Jedrzejowicz, A., Brophy, C., Moxham, J., & Green, M. (1988). *Assessment of Diaphragm Weakness*. American Review Respiratory Disease, Vol. 137 (4), (April 1988): pp. 877-83

Molho, M., Katz, I., Schwartz, E., Shemesh, Y., Sadeh, M., & Wolf, E. (1987). Familial Bilateral Paralysis of Diaphragm. Adult Onset. *Chest*, Vol. 91 (3), (March 1987): pp. 466-7, ISSN 0012-3692

Polkey, M. I., Green, M., & Moxham, J. (1995). Measurement of Respiratory Muscle Strength [Editorial]. *Thorax,* Vol. 50 (11), (November 1995): pp. 1131-5, ISSN 0040-6376

Qureshi, A. (2009). Diaphragm Paralysis. *Seminars in Respiratory Critical Care Medicine*, Vol. 30 (3), (June 2009): pp. 315-20, ISSN 1098-9048

Roussos, C., & Macklem, P.T. (1982). Diaphragmatic Paresis: Pathophysiology, Clinical Features, and Investigation. *N Engl J Med*, Vol. 307 (13), (Sept 1982): pp. 786-97, ISSN 0028-4793

Simansky, D. A., Paley, M., Refaely, Y., & Yellin, A. (2002). Diaphragm Plication Following Phrenic Nerve Injury: a Comparison of Paediatric and Adult Patients. *Thorax*, Vol.57 (7), (July 2002): pp. 613-6, ISSN 0040-6376

Sivan, Y., & Galvis, A. (1990). Early Diaphragmatic Paralysis. In Infants with Genetic Disorders. *Clinical Pediatrics(Phila)*,Vol.29 (3), (March 1990): pp. 169-71, ISSN 0009-9228

Steier, J., Kaul, S., Seymour, J., Jolley, C., Rafferty, G, & Man, W., Lou, Y. M., Roughton, M., Polkey, M. I., & Moxham, J. (2007). The Value of Multiple Tests of Respiratory Muscle Strength. *Thorax*, Vol.62(11), (November 2007): pp.975-80, ISSN 0040-6376

Tarver, R. D., Conces, D. J., Cory, D. A., & Vix, V.A. (1989). Imaging the Diaphragm and its Disorders. *J Thorac Imaging*, Vol. 4 (1), (January 1989): pp. 1-18, ISSN 0883-5993

Tsao, B. E., Ostrovskiy, D. A., Wilbourn, A. J., & Shields, R. W. (2006). Phrenic Neuropathy Due to Neuralgic Amyothrophy. *Neurology*, Vol. 66 (10) (May 2006): pp. 1582-4, ISSN 1526-632X

Versteegh, M. I., Braun, J., Voigt, P.G., Bosman, D. B., Stolk, J., & Rabe, K.F., & Dion, R.A. (2007). Diaphragm Plication in Adult Patients with Diaphragm Paralysis Leads to Long-term Improvement of Pulmonary Function and Level of

Dyspnea. *Eur J Cardiothorac Surg,*Vol. 32 (3) (September 2007): pp.449-56, ISSN 1010-7940

Evidence-Based Prenatal Management in Cases of Congenital Diaphragmatic Hernia

Alex Sandro Rolland Souza
Professor Fernando Figueira Integral Medicine Institute (IMIP)
Recife, Pernambuco
Brazil

1. Introduction

Congenital diaphragmatic hernia (CDH) is the most common defect of the diaphragmatic muscle that separates the thoracic cavity from the abdominal cavity. This malformation allows part of the abdominal structures (intestinal loops, stomach and liver) to herniate into the thoracic cavity, hampering the normal development of the lung and resulting in abnormalities in cardiac function (Santos et al., 2008; Johnson, 2005).

This defect may result in severe repercussions even in the prenatal period, with a high rate of intrauterine or early neonatal mortality, principally due to pulmonary hypoplasia (Santos et al., 2008; Johnson, 2005). Prenatal diagnosis is possible; however, in less severe cases diagnosis may be reached later, beyond the neonatal period at more advanced ages, although this is less common (Santos et al., 2008; Johnson, 2005; Bronshtein et al., 1995; Lewis et al., 1997; Koziarkiewicz & Piaseczna-Piotrowska, 2011).

With the advancement of medical science, survival of these newborn infants has improved; nevertheless mortality remains high (van den Hout et al., 2011; Okuyama et al., 2011). Alternative intrauterine therapies have been studied, with the best results in recent years having been found with the use of fetoscopy (Deprest et al., 2011; Luks, 2011; Peralta et al., 2011). An immense arsenal of treatments for the early neonatal period has also been studied, improving the life of these newborn infants (Henderson-Smart et al., 2011; Mugford et al., 2011; Moyer et al., 2011; Finer & Barrington, 2011).

It is therefore prudent to invest in new diagnostic techniques and therapies for application in the prenatal period in an attempt to permit normal lung development and a consequent improvement in the care provided to these patients.

2. Epidemiology

The incidence of congenital diaphragmatic hernia varies greatly depending on the origin of the data, whether resulting from studies conducted pre- or postnatally or based on surgical studies. In surgical studies, data losses occur due to pregnancy termination, miscarriage, prenatal mortality and immediate neonatal mortality. The neonatal incidence rate is around 1 in 5,000 to 1 in 3,000, whereas the prenatal incidence rate is 1 in 2,000 (Santos et al., 2008; Johnson, 2005).

The most common site of CDH is posterolateral and this malformation is more commonly found in males, in a proportion of 2 to 1. Unilateral CDH is more common than bilateral, with unilateral hernias being more likely to occur on the left side (Santos et al., 2008; Johnson, 2005). A significant association has also been found with other congenital malformations, aneuploidies and genetic syndromes (Santos et al., 2008; Johnson, 2005; Zaiss et al., 2011; Stressig et al., 2011).

3. Anatomy

The diaphragm is the musculotendinous structure interposed between the thoracic and abdominal cavities. It is dome-shaped, its convex upper surface forming the floor of the thoracic cavity and its concave lower surface forming the roof of the abdominal cavity. The muscular portion is located at the peripheral part, being affixed to the lower thoracic wall along its entire circumference, and divided into three portions: sternal, costal and lumbar. The fibers extend from the peripheral part, converging at the center of the muscle and forming the central tendon, where the foramen of the inferior vena cava is situated to the right of the median plane (Fregnani et al., 2005; Sociedade Brasileira de Anatomia, 2001).

The sternal portion of the diaphragm, the smallest part, is attached to the back of the xiphoid process. The fibers of the costal portion are found laterally to the sternal portion. Together, the costal and sternal portions form a small triangular gap on both sides, the base of which faces forwards, with the apex facing backwards towards the central tendon. These gaps are known as the right sternocostal triangle of Morgagni and the left sternocostal triangle of Larrey (Fregnani et al., 2005; Sociedade Brasileira de Anatomia, 2001).

The costal portion comprises the muscular fibers of the lateral region and the anterior portion of the diaphragmatic muscle. The lumbar portion is located in a posterior position, where the esophageal and aortic hiatuses are found. In the posterolateral region, between the costal and lumbar portions, there is a triangular gap on both sides, the base of which is directed downwards to the quadratus lumborum muscle, while the apex is directed upwards to the tendinous center. These gaps are known as the right and left lumbocostal triangles (posterolateral), also known as Bochdalek's triangles (Fregnani et al., 2005; Sociedade Brasileira de Anatomia, 2001).

4. Classification

The diaphragmatic hernia is classified in accordance with the site of the malformation, reflecting its embryologic origin. There are four types of diaphragmatic hernia (Santos et al., 2008; Johnson, 2005):

- Posterolateral defect or Bochdalek hernia, the most common type and responsible for 85-90% of cases detected neonatally. The malformation occurs through the pleuroperitoneal canal and may be unilateral or bilateral. The left side is the more common site, corresponding to 80% of cases. This phenomenon is probably related to the fact that fusion occurs later on the left side than on the right side. Bilateral hernias are the least common, constituting approximately 5% of all cases.
- Parasternal defects or Morgagni hernias are rare, constituting 1-2% of all cases of CDH. They occur in the anterior segment of the diaphragm, between the costal and sternal origins of the organ, on the right.

- Malformations of the septum transversum, located at the midline, occur due to defects in the central tendon of the diaphragm.
- Hiatal hernias are less important clinically. They are the result of a congenitally wide esophageal orifice; however, they do not permit the passage of abdominal organs into the thoracic cavity.

5. Embryology

The diaphragm is formed between the 4th and 12th weeks of pregnancy from the septum transversum, the pleuroperitoneal membrane, the dorsal mesentery of the esophagus and from muscle growth. This structure is totally formed at 8-12 weeks and its fusion is complete before the bowel returns to the abdominal cavity (Arraez-Aybar et al., 2009; Johnson, 2005).

The septum transversum is a mesodermal mass that is formed from the fusion of the third, fourth and fifth myotomes, representing the primordium of the central region of the diaphragm. A caudal migration occurs when the heart descends into the thorax, growing dorsally from the ventrolateral wall of the diaphragm (Arraez-Aybar et al., 2009; Johnson, 2005).

The pleuroperitoneal membrane located midway between the two sides grows ventrally, attaching to the septum transversum anteriorly and to the dorsal mesentery of the esophagus posteriorly, closing parallel to the region of the veins (Arraez-Aybar et al., 2009; Johnson, 2005).

The right hemidiaphragm consolidates earlier than the left, which, together with the position of the liver on the right side, may explain why the Bochdalek hernia is more common on the left side, whereas parasternal hernias are more common on the right, due to the fact that the pericardium protects the left side, hampering the development of hernias on this side (Arraez-Aybar et al., 2009).

6. Etiopathogenesis

No environmental etiological factor has been identified as being potentially responsible for CDH in humans. However, CDH has been induced experimentally with the use of thalidomide, vitamin A deficiency, polybromobiphenyls and nitrofen (Arraez-Aybar et al., 2009). There are reports in the literature that smoking and radiofrequency may constitute possible causes of CDH (Caspers et al., 2010; Yamagami et al., 2011); however, further studies need to be conducted to confirm these hypotheses.

The occurrence of CDH is normally sporadic; nevertheless, familial CDH has already been reported (Narayan et al., 1993). Another study suggested the possibility of alterations in the genome of patients with congenital diaphragmatic hernia, either isolated or non-isolated (Wat et al., 2011). Plenty of evidence of a genetic link in some cases but this is beyond the scope of this chapter.

Two hypotheses have been raised to attempt to explain the origin of diaphragmatic hernias: as a failure in fusion or as a primary defect (Johnson, 2005). It has been suggested that when an abnormality occurs in the development of the diaphragm during the embryonic phase, a malformation occurs in the fusion of the pleuroperitoneal membranes, causing a persistent fault. The abdominal organs then fail to be covered by the peritoneum. Consequently, the hernia sac will also fail to be covered by the peritoneum, as occurs in cases of Bochdalek hernia. This is why it is considered a false hernia (Arraez-Aybar et al., 2009).

On the other hand, in the primary defect, which occurs in the fetal phase when the pleuroperitoneal hiatus has closed but muscle migration is incomplete, the defect is located in the diaphragmatic muscle. Therefore, the increase in abdominal pressure may push the abdominal viscera through the thoracic cavity and consequently the hernia sac will be covered by the peritoneal membrane, as occurs in the case of parasternal hernias. These cases are considered true hernias (Arraez-Aybar et al., 2009). Exceptionally, as the result of diaphragmatic aplasia and of a persistent pericardial-peritoneal shunt, the hernia may occur without a sac, an extremely rare condition known as peritoneopericardial diaphragmatic hernia (Arraez-Aybar et al., 2009; Kessler et al., 1991).

7. Natural history

A diaphragmatic hernia is a congenital malformation occurring in the first trimester of pregnancy; however, the time at which the hernia sac can be identified has yet to be determined. There are well-documented cases in which a prenatal ultrasonography scan performed in the second trimester had been normal but a diagnosis of diaphragmatic hernia was made at a later scan or even at birth (Johnson, 2005; Bronshtein et al., 1995). The time of CDH diagnosis has been evaluated in relation to perinatal prognosis. Survival rates are better in cases diagnosed at birth or in the third trimester compared to cases in which diagnosis is made in the early prenatal phase (Johnson, 2005; Manni et al., 1994). However, when cases diagnosed prenatally were compared with nondiagnostic sonographies (false-negatives), survival was similar in both groups (Johnson, 2005; Lewis et al., 1997). The reason for this herniation occurring earlier or later has yet to be satisfactorily explained in embryological terms (Johnson, 2005).

Pregnancies in which the fetus has a congenital diaphragmatic hernia may be complicated by polyhydramnios, which predisposes the patient to premature delivery. CDH may be associated with other congenital abnormalities, aneuploidies and genetic syndromes, conditions that affect the survival rate (Johnson, 2005).

The necessary conditions for adequate pulmonary development are: adequate intrathoracic space, normal fetal respiratory movement and the presence of a normal amount of amniotic fluid. If one of these conditions is deficient during the canalicular phase of pulmonary development (from the 17th to the 26th weeks of pregnancy), pulmonary hypoplasia will probably occur (Johnson, 2005; Burri, 1984). Therefore, principally as a result of reduced intrathoracic space, pulmonary hypoplasia is common in cases of CDH and constitutes a significant cause of mortality in these patients (Johnson, 2005; Santos, et al., 2008).

8. Prenatal diagnosis

Detailed ultrasonography is the most important method of prenatal diagnosis, since it permits a meticulous evaluation of the CDH and of any associated congenital abnormalities, in addition to following up the condition during pregnancy (Johnson, 2005; Santos, et al.,

2008). Fetal morphological examination by ultrasonography should be performed for the purpose of obtaining the greatest amount of information possible. It is important to determine the site of the lesion, which abdominal organs are inside the thorax, any alterations in amniotic fluid, fetal respiratory pattern, the degree of deviation of the mediastinum and the heart, cardiac compression and pulmonary volume, all of which constitute useful information for evaluating perinatal prognosis and helping define optimal prenatal and postnatal management (Johnson, 2005; Santos, et al., 2008).

CDH may be diagnosed by routine ultrasonography, or in some cases diagnosis is reached when the patient is submitted to a fetal morphological examination performed by a specialist between the 18th and the 20th weeks of pregnancy (Johnson, 2005; Santos, et al., 2008).

Ultrasonographic appearance varies depending on the type of CDH and in accordance with its location (Johnson, 2005; Santos, et al., 2008):

- Identification of the abdominal contents inside the thoracic cavity:
  In cases of left diaphragmatic hernias, the presence of the stomach is viewed in the same plane used to evaluate the four chambers of the heart. When the hernia is located on the left, the stomach, the intestinal loops and the spleen may be found inside the thoracic cavity (Figure 1). If the defect is on the right, it is the liver that may be seen in the fetal thoracic cavity (Figures 2 and 3). It should be emphasized that hernias located on the right side may be diagnosed later in view of the similarity between the echogenic appearance of the hepatic parenchyma and that of the lung.
- Deviation of the mediastinum and heart with cardiac compression (Figures 1 and 2).
- Paradoxical movement of organs during fetal respiratory movement.
- Absence of normal integrity of the diaphragm, as seen on the longitudinal fetal plane.
- Polyhydramnios is generally associated with CDH; however, this condition is rarely seen prior to 24 weeks.

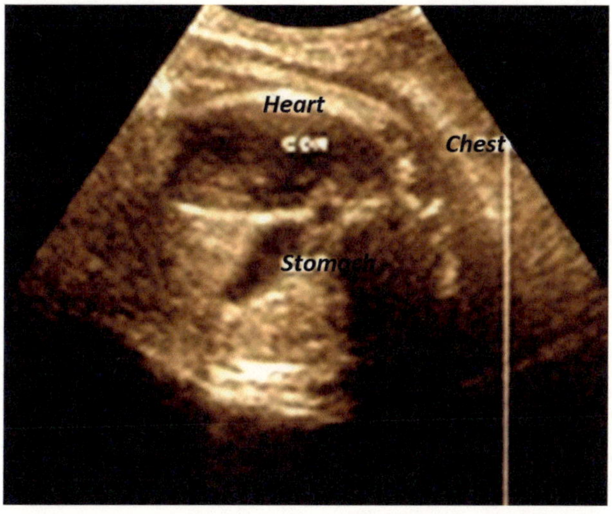

Fig. 1. Ultrasonographic cross-sectional image of the chest. Note the position of the heart deviated to the right and the presence of the stomach (gastric bubble) in the thorax (left diaphragmatic hernia).

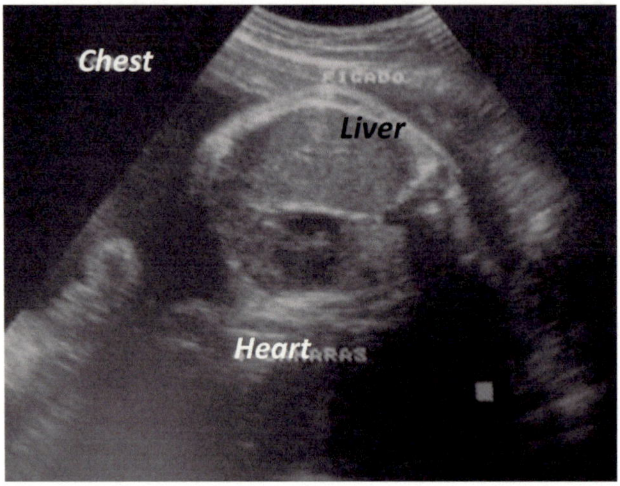

Fig. 2. Ultrasonographic cross-sectional image of the chest. Note the presence of the liver inside the chest, deviating the heart towards the left (right diaphragmatic hernia).

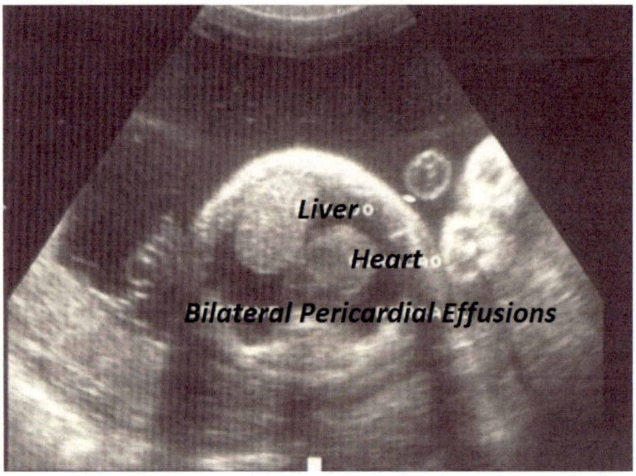

Fig. 3. Ultrasonographic cross-sectional image of the chest. Note the presence of the liver inside the chest, deviating the heart to the left (right diaphragmatic hernia) and the presence of bilateral pericardial effusions.

A normal prenatal ultrasound scan does not guarantee that CDH is not present. The condition may be diagnosed later, still prenatally by ultrasonography or neonatally, even when a previous scan carried out in the second trimester of pregnancy was normal (Bronshtein et al., 1995; Johnson, 2005). [2,3] Many studies have reported a false-positive rate of approximately 50%, with rates being even higher in cases in which the defect has been diagnosed on the right side (Johnson, 2005; Lewis et al., 1997).

At the *Instituto de Medicina Integral Prof. Fernando Figueira* (IMIP), a diagnostic sensitivity of 93%, specificity of 100% and a strong agreement of 96% were found with prenatal ultrasonography performed by fetal medicine specialists compared to perinatal results

(Noronha Neto et al., 2009). It should be emphasized that that study included only patients who were submitted prenatally to ultrasonography in the fetal medicine unit. Patients who had not undergone ultrasonography in this service were excluded from the study. These results are in agreement with findings from other centers reporting diagnosis in almost 100% of cases with an isolated lesion after the 25th week of pregnancy (Bronshtein et al., 1995; Johnson, 2005; Santos et al., 2008). Comparing the data obtained from different centers is difficult, since some centers describe only cases diagnosed prenatally, while others use postnatal data irrespective of the prenatal diagnosis (Johnson, 2005). There have also been literature reports on rare cases in which diagnosis is sometimes made late due to a delayed presentation of CDH symptoms (Koziarkiewicz & Piaseczna-Piotrowska, 2011).

Three-dimensional ultrasonography may also be used for the diagnosis of CDH. Its capacity to measure the volume of fetal structures such as the lung should be assessed in greater depth in order to evaluate fetal prognosis (Prendergast et al., 2011). Likewise, magnetic resonance imaging (MRI) may be used as a complement to conventional ultrasonography; however, its contribution has been more fully evaluated for the assessment of fetal prognosis (Amim et al., 2008; Costa et al., 2011; Souza, 2008).

9. Associated abnormalities

The presence of other congenital abnormalities associated with CDH is common, occurring in around 30-70% of CDH cases diagnosed prenatally (Johnson, 2005; Zaiss et al., 2011) and 40% of cases diagnosed in infancy (Cunniff et al., 1990; Johnson, 2005). Defects of the heart, face, gastrointestinal tract, kidney and neural tube may be associated with CDH (Santos et al., 2008). One study that included 362 fetuses with a diagnosis of CDH found an associated abnormality in 39.5% ofcases. A total of 272 associated abnormalities were diagnosed; however, only 18.4% were diagnosed prenatally. That study reported a wide heterogeneity in these associated malformations, with cardiovascular defects being the most common (Zaiss et al., 2011). An association has also been reported between hypoplasia of the left ventricle and the presence of the liver in the thoracic cavity (Stressig et al., 2011).

In 25 to 34% of cases, there are associated chromosomal abnormalities, trisomy 21 and trisomy 18 being the most common (Johnson, 2005; Santos et al., 2008). Other more complex abnormalities also found include translocations (Johnson, 2005). In such situations, there are other associated structural abnormalities in 73% of cases, the most common being cardiac, skeletal, genitourinary defects and abnormalities of the central nervous system (Johnson, 2005; Santos et al., 2008).

10. Differential diagnosis

Differential diagnosis should be made with other thoracic cystic diseases such as congenital cystic adenomatoid malformation (CCAM) of the lung, bronchogenic cysts, tumors and neurenteric cysts (Santos et al., 2008). At this stage, fetal morphological examination is of crucial importance, and the patient can be submitted to three-dimensional ultrasonography or MRI as a complement to conventional ultrasonography to clarify any remaining doubts.

11. Prenatal conduct

Pregnancies with suspected or confirmed CDH should initially be referred to a specialist perinatal center for confirmatory tests and multidisciplinary follow-up (Santos et al., 2008). At the specialist perinatal center, fetal morphological examination by ultrasonography is used to confirm or refute the initial diagnosis and to provide details of the CDH, or any other abnormalities (Santos et al., 2008).

The following factors regarding the CDH, must be described: the side on which the diaphragmatic hernia is situated, which abdominal organs have been herniated into the thorax, the position of the liver and lung, the degree of deviation of the mediastinum, cardiac compression, the ratio between lung volume and head circumference, estimated lung volume and the volume of amniotic fluid (Johnson, 2005; Santos et al., 2008). Many methods to determine lung volume have been described (Johnson, 2005; Santos et al., 2008) and will be discussed in detail later. The characteristics of fetal respiration have also been evaluated to predict fetal outcome (Badalian et al., 1994; Johnson, 2005).Ultrasound scans should be performed between the 20- 24th weeks of pregnancy, 26- 28th weeks and 32- 34th weeks to evaluate the CDH, any associated abnormalities and to assess fetal growth and vitality (Santos et al., 2008).

Since cardiovascular defects constitute one of the principal abnormalities associated with CDH (Zaiss et al., 2011), a specialist fetal echocardiography is required to evaluate cardiac morphology (Johnson, 2005; Santos et al., 2008).

The parents should be referred for counseling with a multidisciplinary team composed of a fetal medicine specialist, an obstetrician and a neonatologist, as well as a pediatric surgeon specialized in thoracic surgery. Psychological support for the parents is crucial at this time (Johnson, 2005; Santos et al., 2008).

Due to the association of CDH with chromosomal abnormalities, fetal karyotyping is recommended, withe parental consent (Johnson, 2005; Santos et al., 2008). MRI can also be performed to detect the presence or absence of the liver in the thoracic cavity and to help determine fetal outcome (Amim et al., 2008; Costa et al., 2011; Souza, 2008; Terui et al., 2011). The principal causes of death are pulmonary hypoplasia and hypertension (Johnson, 2005; Santos et al., 2008). In an attempt to minimize these complications, Harrison et al. undertook open fetal surgery with disappointing results (Harrison et al., 1993). Intrauterine surgery under these circumstances remains controversial and alternative methods have been proposed such as fetal tracheal occlusion (Harrison et al., 1996). Although theoretically this technique appears promising, further clinical trials still need to be conducted before it can be performed routinely. It is important to emphasize that fetal surgery involves a significant risk of maternal morbidity and should only be undertaken when the expected improvement in fetal survival with this conduct exceeds the risks involved (Johnson, 2005).

More recently, fetal endoscopic tracheal occlusion (FETO) has been used and has proven to be a more viable and safer option. The most common complication is premature rupture of membranes; however, survival rates are apparently higher. Nevertheless, randomized clinical trials must be conducted before FETO can be confirmed as a viable option for increasing survival in these patients. The cases in which FETO may be useful are those involving fetuses with severe single CDH, intrathoracic herniation of the liver and a lung-to-head ratio < 1 (Deprest et al., 2011; Luks, 2011; Peralta et al., 2011; Ruano et al., 2011).

FETO is a technique in which a balloon is introduced for tracheal occlusion through an endoscope with a 1.0 mm optical lens (fetoscopy). This tracheal occlusion permits pulmonary insufflation, thereby increasing intrathoracic pressure, which maintains the abdominal organs outside the thoracic cavity. To perform this procedure, the mother must be under epidural anesthesia and the fetus under intramuscular anesthesia (Ruano et al., 2011).

One study described FETO as a viable alternative for improving neonatal outcome in severe cases of CDH. A higher survival rate (52.9% versus 5.6%; $p<0.01$) and a lower rate of pulmonary hypertension (47.1% versus 88.9%; $p=0.01$) were reported with the use of FETO. There was no statistically significant difference between the groups with respect to gestational age at delivery (35.6 weeks in the FETO group versus 37.5 weeks in the control group); however, it should be emphasized that the sample size was small ($n = 35$ women) (Ruano et al., 2011).

In pregnancies between the 24- 34th weeks, antenatal corticosteroids is administered to accelerate lung maturity in accordance with the risk of prematurity and following routine procedure at each institution (betamethasone or dexamethasone) (Roberts & Dalziel, 2006).

Spontaneous, full-term normal vaginal delivery is preferable; however, labor may be induced (Santos et al., 2008; Souza, 2008). Elective Cesarean section prior to the onset of labor is not recommended except when there is an obstetric indication. In fetuses that have had FETO, Cesarean section is indicated together with ex utero intrapartum therapy (EXIT). This is a Cesarean section in which complete placental circulation is maintained until removal of the balloon and the infant's airways are maintained pervious (Ruano et al., 2011; Nascimento et al., 2007).

12. Prognosis

When there is a confirmed prenatal diagnosis of CDH, prognosis should be established. This is extremely difficult, particularly in view of the increasing advances in perinatology and pediatric surgery, which have contributed towards increasing the perinatal survival rate. Nevertheless, the most important factors in poor prognosis are the presence of associated malformations and the severity of pulmonary hypoplasia and hypertension, mortality rates remaining high in these cases despite the advances in neonatal intensive care with the introduction of extracorporeal membrane oxygenation (ECMO) (Santos et al., 2008).

The probability of survival, as reported in the literature, varies greatly, ranging from 14 to 78% (Johnson, 2005; Okuyama et al., 2011; van den Hout et al., 2011). Various studies have suggested an increase in neonatal survival in patients with CDH resulting from an improvement in management and in medical advances (Okuyama et al., 2011; van den Hout et al., 2011). Nonetheless, it is important to emphasize the heterogeneity of these patients, which in most cases have been conducted in institutions that serve as referral centers.

Therefore, it is important to discuss these survival rates, which should be established in population-based studies (Mah et al., 2011).

The most important indications of poor prognosis, as reported in the literature, are (Johnson, 2005; Santos et al., 2008):

- An association with chromosomal abnormalities and genetic syndromes.
- The presence of associated malformations.
- Suspected pulmonary hypoplasia.
- Large deviation of the mediastinum - defined as a deviation in which, in a cross-sectional plane of the fetal thorax, the heart is found to be entirely in one or the other hemisphere, created by an imaginary line between the sternum and the spine.
- Polyhydramnios, a relatively late manifestation associated with poor prognosis.
- Presence of the liver in the thoracic cavity, which may be diagnosed by MRI.
- Early gestational age at diagnosis.

When the diagnosis is made prior to the 24th week of pregnancy, the prognosis is unfavorable due to the stage of lung development at which the abnormality occurred. In this period, not only are the airways affected, causing pulmonary hypoplasia, but there is also a reduction in the number of blood vessels, resulting in postnatal pulmonary hypertension. In this case, mortality is very high, around 60- 80% (Santos et al., 2008). Therefore, the earlier the prenatal diagnosis, the poorer the prognosis and the lower the probability of perinatal survival (Johnson, 2005; Santos et al., 2008).

Antenatal prediction of pulmonary hypoplasia is important since this diagnosis permits parents to be given appropriate counseling and selection to be carried out of those cases that would benefit from prenatal surgery. However, the issue remains a challenge for specialists in fetal medicine (Santos et al., 2008). The ability to predict perinatal outcome by prenatal ultrasonography when an isolated defect is present is limited, with many studies showing disappointing results (Johnson, 2005).

Various ultrasonographic parameters have been proposed to predict the probability of developing pulmonary hypoplasia. These include thoracic circumference, the calculated difference between the thoracic area and the heart area, lung area, thoracic circumference to abdominal circumference ratio, thoracic area to heart area ratio, the calculated difference between the thoracic area and the heart area to thoracic area ratio, lung-to-thorax transverse area ratio, and the lung-to-head ratio i.e. the ratio between the right lung area and head circumference (Johnson, 2005; Okuyama et al., 2011; Santos et al., 2008; Usui et al., 2011). The area of the right lung is obtained by multiplying the two greatest diameters of the lung. If the lung-to-head ratio is ≤ 1, prognosis is very poor, even if ECMO is instituted at birth. If it is > 1.4, prognosis is more favorable. Values between 1 and 1.4 were associated with a survival rate of 38% and in most cases ECMO was required. The infants who survived had a mean lung-to-head ratio of 1.4 ± 0.33 compared to 1.05 ± 0.3 in those who did not survive (Lipshutz et al., 1997).

Pulmonary blood flow has also been investigated for this purpose. A recent study used Doppler velocimetry of the pulmonary artery to predict prognosis and morbidity in fetuses with a diaphragmatic hernia that had been submitted to FETO. Doppler may also be used to define those fetuses that would benefit from this intrauterine therapy. The study concluded that following therapy, the combination of a relatively greater lung-to-head ratio and better pulmonary tissue perfusion improved the prediction of fetal survival (Cruz-Martinez, et al., 2011).

Therefore, authors suggest that fetuses with a congenital diaphragmatic hernia and a poor prognosis for postnatal treatment can be identified as those in whom part of the liver has been herniated into the thoracic cavity, those in whom diagnosis was made early (prior to the 25th week), those with defects on the left side and the ones with a low lung-to-head ratio (Santos et al., 2008).

It should be emphasized that, in general, all these methods represent efforts to predict pulmonary hypoplasia; however, the reproducibility of these measures has not been considered satisfactory (Johnson, 2005). It should also be noted that pulmonary hypoplasia probably begins prior to the 24th week of pregnancy (at the end of the canalicular phase); therefore, all these parameters are only valid for a diagnosis of pulmonary hypoplasia that is already present and cannot be used to select patients who are candidates for a possible preventive intervention (Johnson, 2005).

MRI can be used to determine prognosis in fetuses with CDH. One study included 12 fetuses with a prenatal diagnosis of CDH who were treated following birth and whose mothers had undergone MRI scanning in the 29th to 37th weeks of pregnancy. The ratio between the intensity of the signal in the lung and the intensity of the signal in the cerebrospinal fluid was calculated by analyzing the region of interest with T2 images. This ratio was found to be significantly higher in the infants who survived compared to those who died, and there was a statistically significant correlation with the duration of endotracheal intubation. The authors suggested that this ratio could be used to evaluate the degree of pulmonary hypoplasia (Terui et al., 2011). MRI has also been used to confirm the presence of the liver in the thoracic cavity, an important prognostic factor (Amim et al., 2008; Souza, 2008).

A study conducted with 153 fetuses with a diagnosis of CDH evaluated the lung-to-head ratio (area of the contralateral lung divided by the circumference of the head) using ultrasonography, while MRI was used to measure lung volume. Measurement of the lung-to-head ratio using ultrasonography provided a good estimate of the fetal lung volume measurement provided by MRI. Additional parameters such as gestational age, the position of the liver and the side of the defect did not increase the accuracy of the calculation of the contralateral lung volume (Sandaite et al., 2011).

Another important point frequently discussed is that prognosis is directly related to neonatal care. One study found that neonatal survival increased from 67% to 88% following implementation of guidelines for the management of patients with CDH. These new guidelines established the administration of nitric oxide in the delivery room, careful ventilation of the newborn infant, fewer criteria for the implementation of ECMO and surgical repair within an appropriate time. It should be emphasized that survival of the patients on ECMO increased from 20% to 82% (Antonoff et al., 2011). Another study conducted with 167 fetuses with CDH diagnosed prenatally also reported an improvement in survival following implementation of guidelines for the management of these patients (van den Hout et al., 2011).

The optimal time to perform surgical correction remains unclear: either after the condition of the infant has been stabilized or immediately within 24 hours. A major randomized, multicenter clinical trial is required to clarify this question (Moyer et al., 2011). Delaying surgery until the infant has been stabilized appears to be associated with better postsurgical outcome; however, this conduct may result in the infant dying prior to surgery in those more severe cases (Johnson, 2005).

In relation to nitric oxide, the available evidence appears to be in favor of the use of inhaled nitric oxide at an initial concentration of 20 ppm for full-term newborns or those born near term with acute hypoxemic respiratory failure; however, there is few randomized clinical trials (RCT) supporting its use in patients with diaphragmatic hernia (Finer & Barrington, 2011).

Modern methods of postnatal management appear to present varying results. ECMO and high-frequency oscillatory ventilation (HFOV) have shown disappointing results, with no great improvement in perinatal survival (Johnson, 2005). Although HFOV plus conventional ventilation has shown results that are similar to those found with ECMO. Up to the present time, there is insufficient evidence, based on RCT, to recommend its use (Henderson-Smart, et al., 2011). It should be noted that ECMO may be associated with long term development problems; therefore, careful follow-up is required (Johnson, 2005).

A meta-analysis made available in the Cochrane library, which includes four randomized clinical trials (n=244), found that the use of ECMO in neonates with severe respiratory failure significantly improved survival, with a lower risk of death prior to discharge from hospital (RR 0.44; 95%CI: 0.31 - 0.61) and a lower risk of death in the first year of life (RR 0.52; 95%CI: 0.37 - 0.73). Nevertheless, there is insufficient evidence for its use in patients with CDH (Mugford et al., 2011).

13. References

[1] Amim, B.; Werner Jr, H.; Daltro, P.D.; Antunes, E.; Fazecas, T.; Rodrigues, L.; Guerra, F.; Marchiori, E.; Gaspareto, E.L. & Domingues, R.C. (2008). O valor da ultra-sonografia e da ressonância magnética fetal na avaliação das hérnias diafragmáticas. *Radiol Bras*, Vol.41, No.1, pp.1-6.

[2] Antonoff, M.B.; Hustead, V.A.; Groth, S.S. & Schmeling, D.J. (2011). Protocolized management of infants with congenital diaphragmatic hernia: effect on survival. *J Pediatr Surg*, Vol.46, No.1, pp.39-46.

[3] Arraez-Aybar, L.A.; Gonzalez-Gomez, C.C. & Torres-Garcia, A.J. (2009). Morgagni-Larrey parasternal diaphragmatic hernia in the adult. *Rev Esp Enferm Dig*, Vol.101, No.5, pp.357-66.

[4] Badalian, S.S.; Fox, H.E.; Chao, C.R.; Timor-Tritsch, I.E. & Stolar, C.J. (1994). Fetal breathing characteristics and postnatal outcome in cases of congenital diaphragmatic hernia. *Am J Obstet Gynecol*, Vol.171, No.4, pp.790-6.

[5] Bronshtein, M.; Lewit, N.; Sujov, P.O.; Makhoul, I.R. & Blazer S. (1995). Prenatal diagnosis of congenital diaphragmatic hernia: timing of visceral herniation and outcome. *Prenat Diagn*, Vol.15, No.8, pp.695-8.

[6] Burri, P.H. (1984). Fetal and post-natal development of the lung. *Ann R Physiol*, Vol.46, pp.R617-28.

[7] Caspers, K.M.; Oltean, C.; Romitti, P.A.; Sun, L.; Pober, B.R.; Rasmussen, A.S.; Yang, W.; Druschel, C. & National Birth Defects Prevention Study. (2010). Maternal periconceptional exposure to cigarette smoking and alcohol consumption and congenital diaphragmatic hernia. *Birth Defects Res A Clin Mol Teratol*, Vol.88, No.12, pp.1040-9.

[8] Costa, F.; Kaganov, H.; O'Mahony, E.; Ng, J.; Fink, A.M. & Palma-Dias, R. (2011). Diagnosis of diaphragmatic hernia with associated congenital lung lesions: contribution of fetal MRI. *Fetal Diagn Ther*, Vol.29, No.1, pp.:111-5.

[9] Cruz-Martinez, R.; Hernandez-Andrade, E.; Moreno-Alvarez, O.; Done, E.; Deprest, J. & Gratacos, E. (2011). Prognostic value of pulmonary Doppler to predict response to tracheal occlusion in fetuses with congenital diaphragmatic hernia. *Fetal Diagn Ther* Vol.29, No.1, pp.18-24.

[10] Cunniff, C.; Jones, K.L. & Jones, M.C. (1990). Patterns of malformations in children with congenital diaphragmatic defects. *J Pediatr*, Vol.116, No.2, pp.258-61.

[11] Deprest, J.; Nicolaides, K.; Done, E.; Lewi, P.; Barki, G.; Largen, E.; DeKoninck, P.; Sandaite, I.; Ville, Y.; Benachi, A.; Jani, J.; Amat-Roldan, I.; Gratacos, E. (2011). Technical aspects of fetal endoscopic tracheal occlusion for congenital diaphragmatic hernia. *J Pediatr Surg*, Vol.46, No.1, pp.22-32.

[12] Finer, N. & Barrington, K.J. (2011). Nitric oxide for respiratory failure in infants born at or near term. Cochrane Database of Systematic Reviews. In: *The Cochrane Library*, Issue 08, Art. No. CD000399. DOI: 10.1002/14651858.CD000399.pub1.

[13] Fregnani, J.H.T.G.; Macéa, J.R. & Barros, M.D. (2005). Cirurgia no hiato esofágico: a identificação correta das estruturas anatômicas. *Rev Bras Videocir*, Vol.3, No.1, pp.15-20.

[14] Harrison, M.R.; Adzick, N.S. & Flake, A.W. (1993). Congenital diaphragmatic hernia: an unsolved problem. *Semin Pediatr Surg*, Vol.2, No.2. pp.109-12.

[15] Harrison, M.R.; Adzick, N.S. & Flake, A.W. (1996). Correction of congenital diaphragmatic hernia in utero: VIII. Response of the hypoplastic lung to tracheal occlusion. *J Pediatr Surg*, Vol.31, pp.1339-48.

[16] Henderson-Smart, D.J.; De Paoli, A.G.; Clark, R.H. & Bhuta, T. (2011). High frequency oscillatory ventilation versus conventional ventilation for infants with severe pulmonary dysfunction born at or near term. Cochrane Database of Systematic Reviews. In: *The Cochrane Library*, Issue 08, Art. No. CD002974. DOI: 10.1002/14651858.CD002974.pub.

[17] Johnson, P. (2005). Malformações torácicas, In: *Medicina Fetal Fundamentos e Prática Clínica [Fetal Medicine: Basic Science and Clinical Practice]* (1st Ed), Rodeck, C.H. & Whittle, M.J, (Editors), pp. 651-63, Revinter, ISBN 978-85-7309-857-0, Rio de Janeiro, Brasil.

[18] Kessler, R.; Pett, S. & Wernly, J. (1991). Peritoneopericardial diaphragmatic hernia discovered at coronary bypass operation. *Ann Thorac Surg*; 52: 562-3.

[19] Koziarkiewicz, M. & Piaseczna-Piotrowska, A. (2011). Pózna manifestacja wrodzonej przepukliny przeponowej - opis przypadku [Late manifestation of congenital diaphragmatic hernia - case report]. *Med Wieku Rozwoj*, Vol.15, No.1, pp.106-9.

[20] Lewis, D.A.; Reickert, C.; Bowserman, R.; Hirschl, R.B. (1997). Prenatal ultrasonography frequently fails to diagnose congenital diaphragmatic hernia. *J Pediatr Surg*, Vol.32, No.2, pp.352-6.

[21] Lipshutz, G.S.; Albanese, C.T.; Feldestein, V.A.; Jennings, R.W.; Housley, H.T.; Beech, R.; Farrell, J.A. & Harrison MR. (1997). Prospective analysis of lung-to-head ratio predicts survival for patients with prenatally diagnosed congenital diaphragmatic hernia. *J Pediatr Surg*, Vol.32, No.11, pp.1634-6.

[22] Luks, F.I. (2011). New and/or improved aspects of fetal surgery. *Prenat Diagn*, Vol.31, No.3, pp.252-8.

[23] Mah, V.K.; Chiu, P. & Kim, P.C. (2011). Are we making a real difference? Update on 'hidden mortality' in the management of congenital diaphragmatic hernia. *Fetal Diagn Ther*, Vol.29, No.1, pp.40-5.

[24] Manni, M.; Heydanus, R.; Den-Hollander, N.S.; Tewart, P.A.; De Vogelaere, C. & Wladimiroff, J.W. (1994). Prenatal diagnosis of congenital diaphragmatic hernia: a retrospective analysis of 28 cases. *Prenat Diagn*, Vol.14, pp.187-90.

[25] Moyer, V.A.; Moya, F.R.; Tibboel, D.; Losty, P.D.; Nagaya, M. & Lally, K.P. (2011). Late versus early surgical correction for congenital diaphragmatic hernia in newborn infants. Cochrane Database of Systematic Reviews. In: *The Cochrane Library*, Issue 08, Art. No. CD001695. DOI: 10.1002/14651858.CD001695.pub3.

[26] Mugford, M.; Elbourne, D. & Field D. (2011). Extracorporeal membrane oxygenation for severe respiratory failure in newborn infants. Cochrane Database of Systematic Reviews. In: *The Cochrane Library*, Issue 08, Art. No. CD001340. DOI: 10.1002/14651858.CD001340.pub1.

[27] Narayan, H.C.R.; Barrow, M.; Mckeever, P. & Neale, E. (1993). Familial congenital diaphragmatic hernia: prenatal diagnosis, management and outcome. *Prenat Diagn*, Vol.13, No.10, pp.893-901.

[28] Nascimento, G.C.; Souza, A.S.R.; Lima, M.M.S.; Guerra, G.V.; Meneses, J.A.; Cardoso, A.S. & Azevedo, K.S. (2007). Estratégia de conduta intraparto no teratoma cervical congênito: procedimento EXIT (Tratamento extra-útero intraparto). *Act Med Port*, Vol.20, pp.221-7.

[29] Noronha Neto, C.; Souza, A.S.R.; Moraes Filho, O.B. & Noronha, A.M.B. (2009). Validação do diagnóstico ultrassonográfico de anomalias fetais em centro de referência. *Rev Assoc Med Bras*, Vol.55, No.5, pp.541-6.

[30] Okuyama, H.; Kitano, Y.; Saito, M.; Usui, N.; Morikawa, N.; Masumoto, K.; Takayasu, H.; Nakamura, T.; Ishikawa, H.; Kawataki, M.; Hayashi, S.; Inamura, N.; Nose, K. & Sago, H. (2011). The Japanese experience with prenatally diagnosed congenital diaphragmatic hernia based on a multi-institutional review. *Pediatr Surg Int*, Vol.27, No.4, pp.373-8.

[31] Peralta, C.F.; Sbragia, L.; Bennini, J.R.; Braga, F.A.A.; Sampaio, R.M.; Machado, R.I.R. & Barini, R. (2011). Fetoscopic endotracheal occlusion for severe isolated diaphragmatic hernia: initial experience from a single clinic in Brazil. *Fetal Diagn Ther*, Vol.29, No.1, pp.71-7.

[32] Prendergast, M.; Rafferty, G.F.; Davenport, M.; Persico, N.; Jani, J.; Nicolaides, K. & Greenough, A. (2011). Three-dimensional ultrasound fetal lung volumes and infant respiratory outcome: a prospective observational study. *BJOG*, Vol.118, No.5, pp.608-14.

[33] Roberts, D. & Dalziel, S. (2006). Antenatal corticosteroids for accelerating fetal lung maturation for women at risk of preterm birth. *Cochrane Database Syst Rev*; 3:CD004454.

[34] Ruano, R.; Duarte, A.S.; Pimenta, E.J.; Takashi, E.; da Silva, M.M.; Tannuri, U. & Zugaib, M. (2011). Comparison between fetal endoscopic tracheal occlusion using a 1.0-mm fetoscope and prenatal expectant management in severe congenital diaphragmatic hernia. *Fetal Diagn Ther*, Vol.29, No.1, pp.64-70.

[35] Sandaite, I.; Claus, F.; De Keyzer, F.; Done, E.; Van Mieghem, T.; Gucciardo, L.; DeKoninck, P.; Jani, J.; Cannie, M. & Deprest, J.A. (2011). Examining the relationship between the lung-to-head ratio measured on ultrasound and lung volumetry by magnetic resonance in fetuses with isolated congenital diaphragmatic hernia. *Fetal Diagn Ther*, Vol.29, No.1, pp.80-7.

[36] Santos, L.C.; Figueiredo, S.R.; Souza, A.S.R. & Marques M. (2008). *Medicina Fetal* (1st Ed), Medbook, ISBN 978-85-99977-19-4, Rio de Janeiro, Brasil.

[37] Sociedade Brasileira de Anatomia. (2001). *Terminologia Anatômica*. Terminologia Anatômica Internacional (1st Ed.), Manole, São Paulo, Brasil.

[38] Souza, A.S.R. (2008). O valor da ultra-sonografia e da ressonância magnética fetal na avaliação das hérnias diafragmáticas. *Radiol Bras*, Vol.41, No.3, pp.VII-VIII.

[39] Stressig, R.; Fimmers, R.; Eising, K.; Gembruch, U. & Kohl, T. (2011). Intrathoracic herniation of the liver ('liver-up') is associated with predominant left heart hypoplasia in human fetuses with left diaphragmatic hernia. *Ultrasound Obstet Gynecol*, Vol.37, No.3, pp.272-6.

[40] Terui, K.; Omoto, A.; Osada, H.; Hishiki, T.; Saito, T.; Sato, Y; Nakata, M.; Komatsu, S.; Ono, S. & Yoshida, H. (2011). Prediction of postnatal outcomes in congenital diaphragmatic hernia using MRI signal intensity of the fetal lung. *J Perinatol*, Vol.31, No.4, pp.269-73.

[41] Usui, N.; Kitano, Y.; Okuyama, H.; Saito, M.; Morikawa, N.; Takayasu, H.; Nakamura, T.; Hayashi, S.; Kawataki, M.; Ishikawa, H.; Nose, K.; Inamura, N.; Masumoto, K. & Sago, H. (2011). Reliability of the lung to thorax transverse area ratio as a predictive parameter in fetuses with congenital diaphragmatic hernia. *Pediatr Surg Int*, Vol.27, No.1, pp.39-45.

[42] van den Hout, L.; Schaible, T.; Cohen-Overbeek, T.E.; Hop, W.; Siemer, J.; van de Ven, K.; Wessel, L.; Tibboel, D. & Reiss, I. (2011). Actual outcome in infants with congenital diaphragmatic hernia: the role of a standardized postnatal treatment protocol. *Fetal Diagn Ther*, Vol.29, No.1, pp.55-63.

[43] Zaiss, I.; Kehl, S.; Link, K.; Neff, W.; Schaible, T.; Sütterlin, M. & Siemer, J. (2011). Associated malformations in congenital diaphragmatic hernia. *Am J Perinatol,* Vol.28, No.3, pp.211-8.

[44] Yamagami, T.; Yoshimatsu, R.; Matsushima, S.; Tanaka, O.; Miura, H. & Nishimura, T. (2011). Diaphragmatic hernia after radiofrequency ablation for hepatocellular carcinoma. *Cardiovasc Intervent Radiol,* Vol.34, No.Suppl 2, pp.S175-7.

[45] Wat, M.J.; Veenma, D.; Hogue, J.; Holder, A.M.; Yu, Z.; Wat, J.J.; Hanchard, N.; Shchelochkov, O.A.; Fernandes, C.J.; Johnson, A.; Lally, K.P.; Slavotinek, A.; Danhaive, O.; Schaible, T.; Cheung, S.W.; Rauen, K.A.; Tonk, V.S.; Tibboel, D.; de Klein, A. & Scott, D.A. (2011). Genomic alterations that contribute to the development of isolated and non-isolated congenital diaphragmatic hernia. *J Med Genet,* Vol.48, No.5, pp.299-307.

Section 2

Diagnosis and Investigation of Congenital Diaphragmatic Hernia

4

Rare Congenital Diaphragmatic Defects

Man Mohan Harjai
Surgical Division Army Hospital (Research and Referral), New Delhi
India

1. Introduction

Congenital diaphragmatic hernia (CDH) is a developmental defect of the diaphragm that allows abdominal viscera to herniate into the chest. The reported incidence of CDH is estimated to be between 1 in 2000 to 5000 births. Defects are more common on the left side, with approximately 80% being left sided and 20% right sided. Bilateral CDH defects are rare and have a high incidence of associated anomalies.

CDH is thought to represent a sporadic developmental anomaly, although a number of familial cases have been reported. The cause of a CDH is unknown. As with other embryopathies there is increasing evidence that CDH may be due to the exposure of genetically predisposed or susceptible individuals to environmental factors. The embryologic development of the diaphragm remains incompletely understood and involves multiple, complex cellular and tissue interactions. The fully developed diaphragm is derived from four distinct components: (a) the anterior central tendon forms from the septum transversum, (b) the dorsolateral portions form from the pleuroperitoneal membranes, (c) the dorsal crura evolve from the esophageal mesentery, and (d) the muscular portion of the diaphragm develops from the thoracic intercostal muscle groups. Failure of normal closure of the pleuroperitoneal canal in the developing embryo and delay or failure of muscular fusion results to development of diaphragmatic defect and herniation of abdominal contents. Abdominal contents herniate and compress the ipsilateral developing lung. The volume of herniated contents may be small or large enough to contain most of the gut, spleen, or liver. Because herniation occurs during a critical period of lung development when bronchial and pulmonary artery branching occurs, lung compression by the herniated bowel results in pulmonary hypoplasia. In addition, arterial branching is reduced and there is muscular hyperplasia of the pulmonary arterial tree, resulting in pulmonary hypertension.

Affected neonates usually present in the first few hours of life with respiratory distress that may be mild or so severe as to be incompatible with life. Infants with CDH most often develop respiratory distress in the first few hours or days of life. The spectrum of presentation can vary from acute, severe respiratory distress at birth, which is common, to minimal or no symptoms and they may present late which is less common (beyond the neonatal period) and represents true diagnostic challenge. Diagnosis of the defect is difficult. Symptoms are non-specific and can be misleading.

2. Types of diaphragmatic defects

Various types of Diaphragmatic defects include (a) paravertebral type or posterolateral type (Bochdalek type) (80%) (b) parasternal type (in the anterior foramen of Morgagni) (c) diaphragmatic eventration, (d) central diaphragmatic hernia (septum transversum) and (e) diaphragmatic agenesis (1/250 000 births). The central CDH occurs in the midline of the septum transversum and accounts for 1 to 2% of the total cases of CDH.

3. Anterior diaphragmatic hernia of Morgagni

The anterior diaphragmatic hernia of Morgagni is located anteromedially on either side of the junction of the septum transversum and the thoracic wall. Morgagni hernia is a rare malformation (2 - 3% of diaphragmatic hernias). This hernia is usually asymptomatic in children. The rarity, as well as the vague and nonspecific presentations, contributes to the delay in diagnosis. Commonly, the presentation in the pediatric age group is that of recurrent chest infection and rarely with gastrointestinal symptoms. The variable clinical picture results in a considerable diagnostic challenge. Up to 5% of cases are incidentally identified in adults undergoing studies for other reasons. Physicians caring for these patients should be aware of this, and a high index of suspicion is recommended to obviate delay in diagnosis with its associated morbidity. Presentation of the Morgagni hernia with obstruction had been reported in adult but not in children (1). Diagnosis is usually by chest radiograph in 2 planes or CT scan. The optimal method of surgical repair is not known due to the rarity of this condition. The surgical approach may be either transabdominal or thoracic. The surgical repair is indicated even in asymptomatic patients. There are increasing reports about the role of minimally invasive approach. The recurrence is low with an excellent prognosis. (2). Morgagni hernia should be strongly considered in patients with Down's syndrome admitted repeatedly for chest infections. (3). Sternal clefts are rare chest wall anomalies which may occur in isolation or in association with cardiac, pericardial, and anterior diaphragmatic defects (4). The intrathoracic herniation of liver through Morgagni hernia may compressed the right chambers of the heart in a newborn causing cardiac compression (tamponade) resulting in a diagnostic dilemma (5). The autopsy findings in a newborn revealed multiple uncommon anomalies associated with diaphragmatic defects. The baby had bilateral diaphragmatic agenesis associated with right pulmonary hypoplasia, left pulmonary agenesis, multiple cardiac abnormalities and gallbladder agenesis, which is a very rare entity and incompatible with life (6).

4. Congenital diaphragmatic eventration

Congenital diaphragmatic eventration is defined as the abnormal elevation of the diaphragm and is characterized by muscular aplasia, resulting from impaired ingrowth of muscle fibres into the diaphragm during the first trimester. The abnormally elevated diaphragm may compress the ipsilateral lung, and with respiratory effort the mediastinum may shift towards the normal side. The congenital form may be indistinguishable from a diaphragmatic hernia with a sac, and symptoms are usually similar. Diagnosis is usually made on fluoroscopy or ultrasound examination of the chest. In such cases, the diaphragm moves paradoxically with respiratory motion. This paradoxic movement may be so marked that it results in severe compromise of gas exchange. A small eventration may be left untreated (7). Repair is indicated when a large functional deficit in the function of the ipsilateral lung on ventilation/perfusion studies is found in an apparently asymptomatic patient. In such cases, the compressed lung will not grow well. For the same reason, a large eventration should be repaired even when asymptomatic. If the defect is large, it may not be possible to repair it by direct approximation with nonabsorbable interrupted 2-0 sutures. The use of prerenal fascia, rib structures, the latissimus dorsi muscle, rotational muscle flaps from the thoraco-abdominal wall and prosthetic patches is recommended in difficult and wide gap hernias. Repair may be performed either through the abdomen or the chest either as an open procedure or laparoscopically.

Congenital anomalies in the position or attachment of proximal portion of alimentary tube occur as a part of general transposition of the viscera. Situs inversus totalis is a rare, congenital condition that is characterized by the development of the thoracic and abdominal viscera in a mirror image to their normal orientation but isolated dextrogastria is the rarest of all visceral transpositions. Isolated dextrogastria is a very rare congenital anomaly in which the stomach is right-sided while the intestines, the organs in the chest, and the other organs in the abdomen are in normal situs. This rare anomaly can coexists with eventration of the right hemidiaphragm, creating further confusion. These rare combinations often present difficulties in diagnosis which may lead to inappropriate treatment. It may simulate abscess, right-sided hiatal hernia, pleural effusion, pneumonia or other pathology at the right base. The importance of recognising the spectrum of situs anomalies is because the altered anatomy associated with these anomalies may result in misdiagnosis. At times it is difficult to distinguish preoperatively between eventration of diaphragm and congenital diaphragmatic hernia with a sac in a newborn [8].

The association of isolated asymptomatic dextrogastria (Fig 1, 2) with eventration of the right hemidiaphragm creates a diagnostic dilemma, delay in diagnosis and management in such cases (9). Evaluation with contrast in such cases is often suboptimal and MRI may help in these neonates and infants depicting the anomaly without radiation risk to the child [10]. Gastric volvulus of the right sided stomach in an infant with eventration of right hemi-diaphragm associated with malrotation is reported in the literature with its diagnostic dilemmas [11]. The diagnostic uncertainty could only be solved at laparotomy in such cases. However, this clinical entity should be taken into account in the differential diagnosis of children with respiratory distress and GI disturbances.

5. Congenital diaphragmatic hernia

The late presentation of the congenital diaphragmatic hernia (CDH) with subtle symptoms of recurrent colicky pain abdomen or respiratory distress are sometime misleading and the first requisite for the diagnosis of a congenital diaphragmatic hernia (CDH) in late presenters is a high index of suspicion. These types of cases require evaluation with X-Ray Chest, contrast study of gut and if required CT scan of chest. (Fig 3 to 9). The lack of typical clinical presentation in cases of late presenting CDH leads to delayed diagnosis of the defect (12). Cystic lesions or masses in the lower lung fields should suggest the possibility of a CDH with herniated abdominal content at any age.

Congenital diaphragmatic hernias should be included in the differential diagnosis of apparent lower lobe pneumonias in all children below a month of age (13). In a series of 12

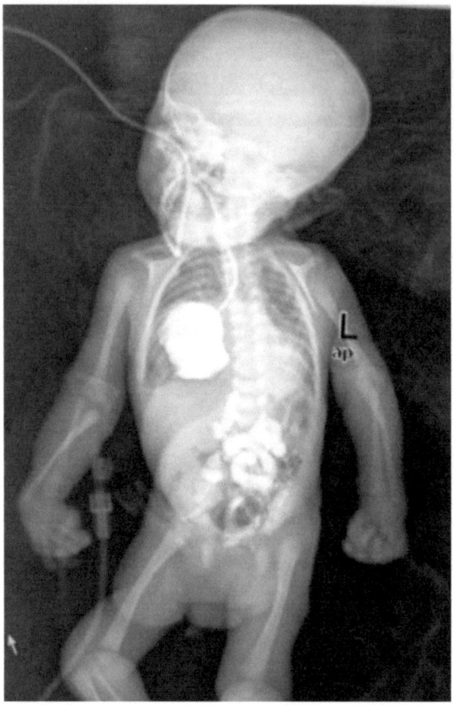

Fig. 1 Contrast radiograph showing stomach lying on the right side of chest while all other viscera's are normally placed in a case of right eventration of diaphragm with isolated dextrogastria.

patients of delayed presentation of CDH, authors found that most of the patients presented with recurrent chest infections (14). However in another observation the authors noticed that the gastrointestinal problems were more common in left-sided hernias, whereas respiratory symptoms predominated in right-sided lesions in late-onset CDH (15). The authors from Egypt concluded that the late-presenting CDH should be included in the differential diagnosis of any child with recurrent non specific respiratory or gastrointestinal symptoms associated with an abnormal chest X-ray film and GI contrast studies should be a part of the diagnostic work-up of these patients (16. 17, 18, 19, 20)). However, when a diagnosis of CDH has been established, albeit asymptomatic, it must be promptly treated surgically in order to prevent complications, such as strangulation or bowel perforation, and thus avert a potentially fatal outcome. The endoscopic approach of late-presenting Morgagni and Bochdalek CDH is also a safe alternative in expert hands (21). In an interesting case report of right-sided Bochdalek hernia with a right intrathoracic stomach and organo-axial torsion which was misdiagnosed initially, and was treated as a case of hyperactive airway disease. The child was operated by right thoracotomy, excision of the hernia sac that contained the stomach, greater omentum and part of the liver was done and reduction of the viscera into the abdominal cavity with simple closure of the diaphragmatic defect was carried out (22). Thus the late presentation has been associated with varied manifestations, hence proper clinical evaluation, a high index of suspicion and adequate management, which includes imaging and surgery after stabilization, gives excellent results in such cases.

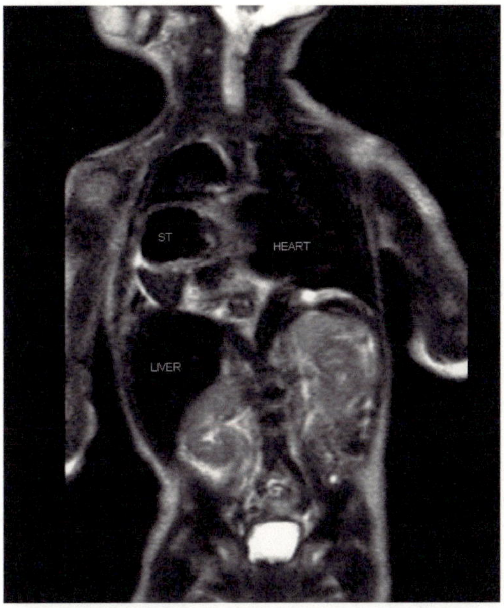

Fig. 2 MRI reconstruction of newborn revealed stomach (ST) lying on the right side of chest above the liver while all other viscera's are normally placed.

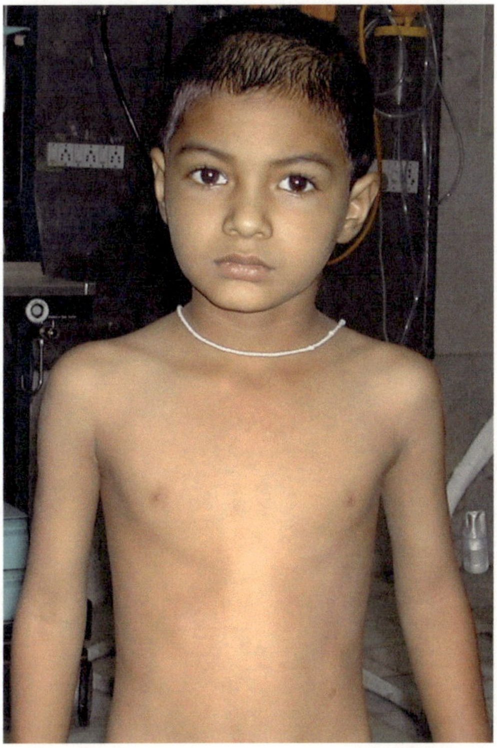

Fig. 3. Clinical photograph of the 7 year old male boy presented with history of recurrent colicky pain abdomen and respiratory distress.

The rare cases of unilateral diaphragmatic defects (agenesis) are also reported in the literature, which may remain undetected till adult life (23). Even in a rare combination the right congenital diaphragmatic hernia and an anorectal malformation coexisted in a neonate (24). A combination of two rare birth defects i.e. oculocutaneous albinism and a right-sided congenital diaphragmatic hernia was reported in a male Asian baby in the literature (25). A rare case of left pulmonary agenesis associated with congenital diaphragmatic hernia and congenital heart disease in a 2-year-old child with pulmonary hypertension is described in the literature (26). In 3 neonates complete absence of pericardium and ectopic liver has been described associated with congenital diaphragmatic hernia (27).

There are various atypical anomalies associated with Morgagni diaphragmatic defects presenting late, with less than 300 adult cases reported in the literature. In a 90-year-old woman, during her evaluation for a lung mass, the herniation of the liver through the foramen of Morgagni was detected on PET/CT scan (28). In a rare association Niramis R et al reported a 2-year-and-2-month-old boy with Down syndrome who had bilateral Morgagni and left Bochdalek hernias with hernial sacs in all of the diaphragmatic defects (29).

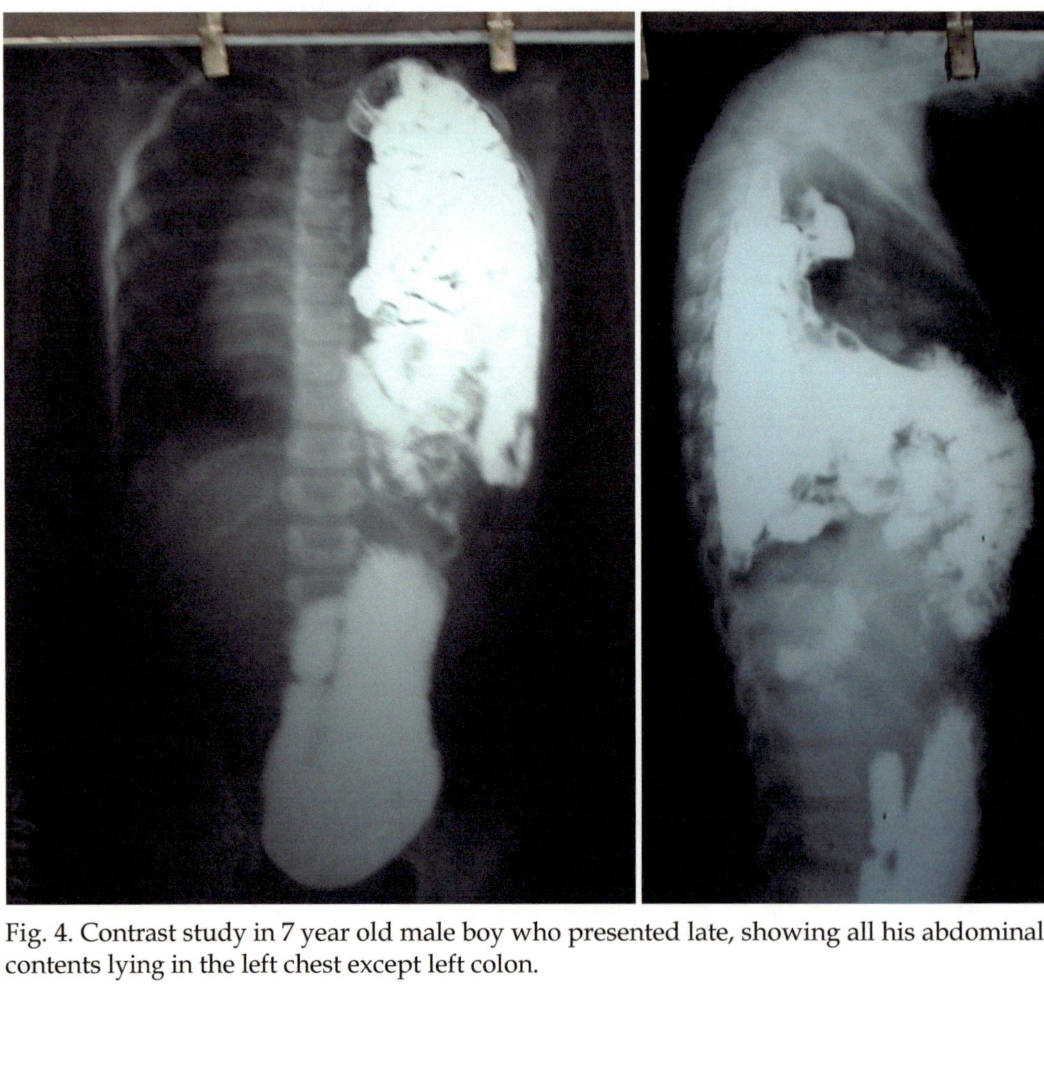

Fig. 4. Contrast study in 7 year old male boy who presented late, showing all his abdominal contents lying in the left chest except left colon.

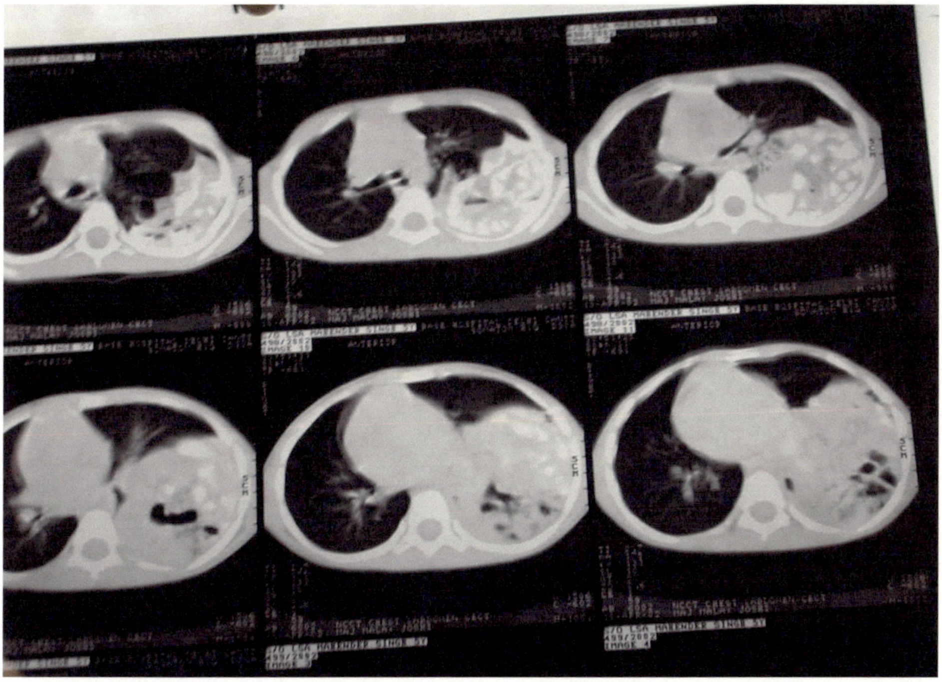

Fig. 5. CT scan of chest showing gut contents in the left chest.

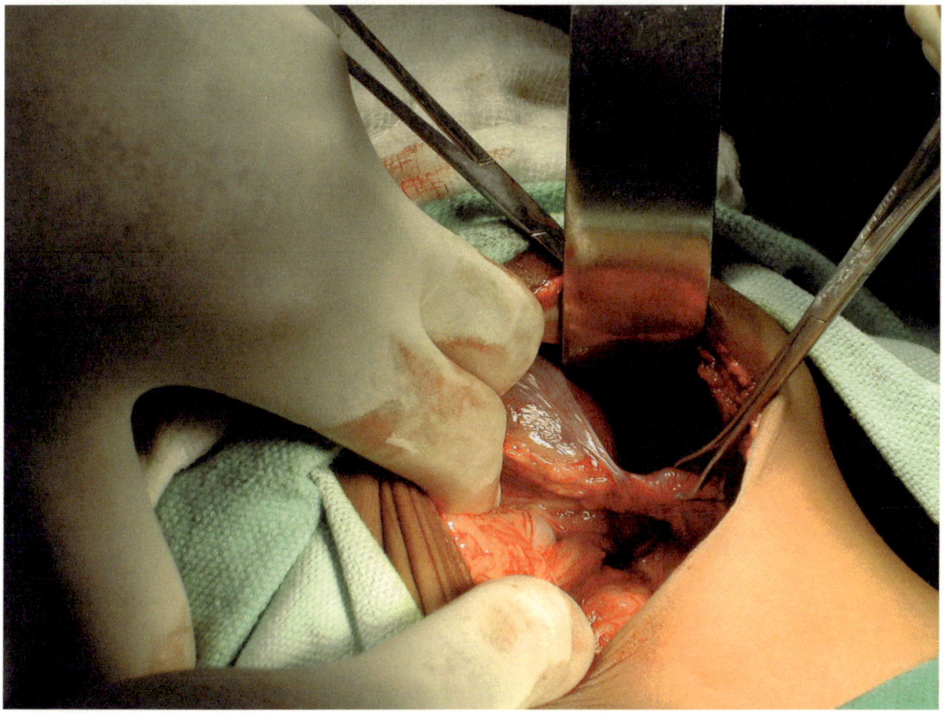

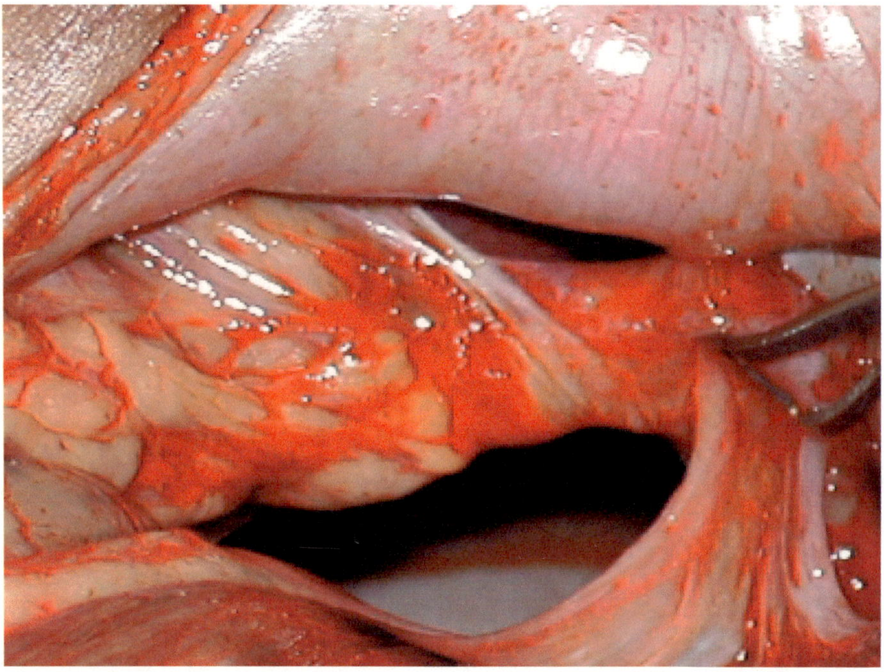

Fig. 6. Operative photographs showing diaphragmatic defect on the left side in the same boy who presented late at age of 7 year.

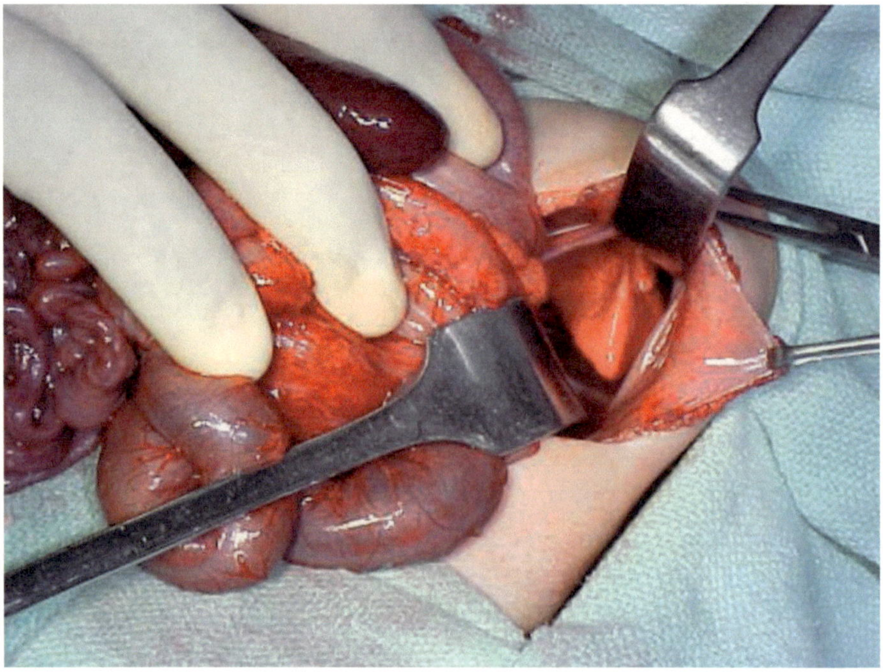

Fig. 7. Operative photograph of a case of Congenital Diaphragmatic Hernia, showing reduced contents and a small hypoplastic lung peeping through defect.

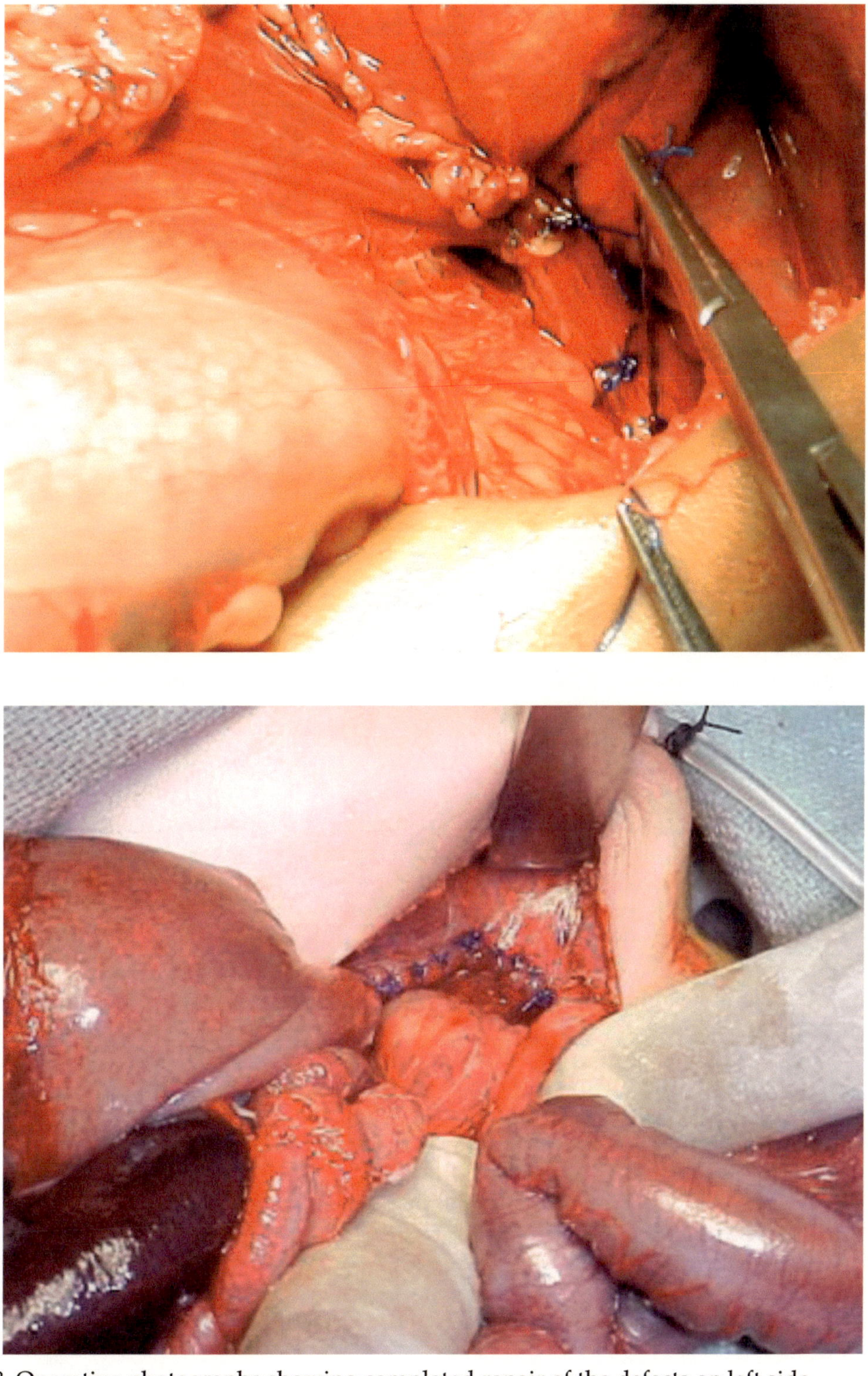

Fig. 8. Operative photographs showing completed repair of the defects on left side.

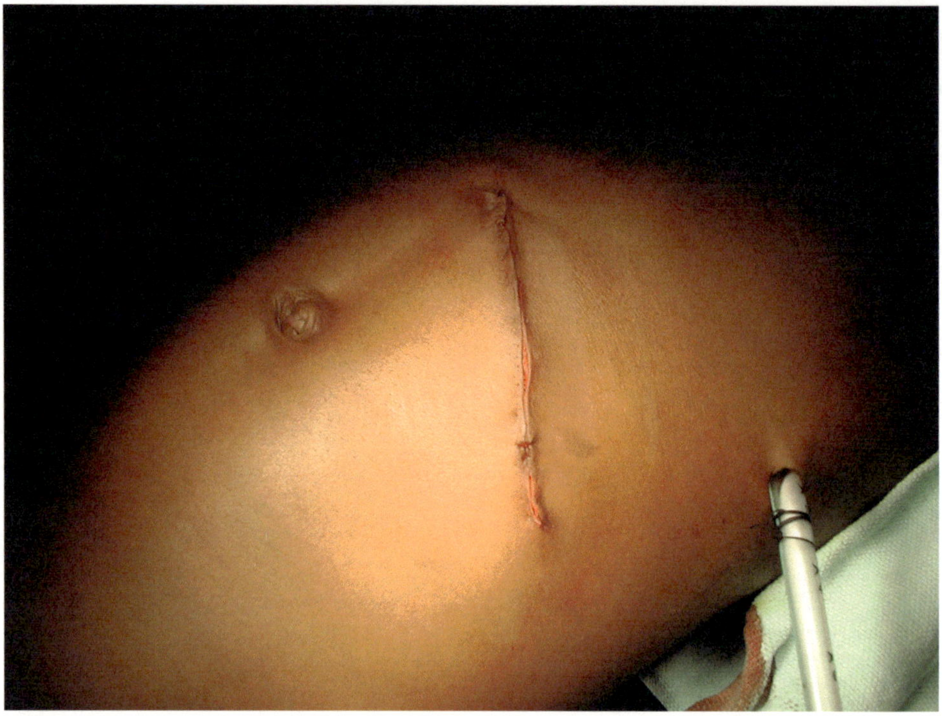

Fig. 9. Final photograph after repair of CDH in a boy who presented late, showing abdominal distension due to filling of abdominal cavity by contents from the chest cavity.

6. Summary

The rare congenital diaphragmatic defects are always posing a diagnostic challenge and require a very high index of clinical suspicion. Symptoms are always non-specific and can be misleading. The diagnosis of these defects is problematical. The rarity, as well as the vague and nonspecific presentations, contributes to the delay in diagnosis. At times the diagnostic uncertainty could only be solved at laparotomy in such cases. All such cases can be managed with open or minimal invasive surgery, once optimally stabilized. The outcome in such cases always depends on the presence or absence of associated other congenital anomalies.

7. References

Gangopadhyay AN, Upadhyaya VD, Gupta DK, Sharma SP. Obstructed Morgagni's hernia. Indian J Pediatr. 2007; 74: 1109-10

Nasr A, Fecteau A. Foramen of Morgagni hernia: presentation and treatment. Thorac Surg Clin. 2009; 19: 463-8.

Jetley NK, Al-Assiri AH, Al-Helal AS, Al-Bin Ali AM. Down's syndrome as a factor in the diagnosis, management, and outcome in patients of Morgagni hernia. J Pediatr Surg. 2011 46: 636-9.

Slone T, Emil S, Meissner N, Behjatnia B, Fairbanks T, Romansky S. Sternal cleft, Morgagni hernia, and ectopic liver: a unique chest wall anomaly. J Pediatr Surg. 2007; 42: 2132-5.

S Breinig, Paranon S, Le Mandat A, Galinier P, Dulac Y, Acar P. Morgagni hernia causing cardiac tamponade. Arch Pediatr. 2010; 17:1465-8.

Karadeniz L, Guven S, Atay E, Ovali F, Celayir A. Bilateral diaphragmatic defect and associated multiple anomalies. J Chin Med Assoc. 2009; 72:163-5.

Sandstrom CK, Stern EJ. Diaphragmatic hernias: a spectrum of radiographic appearances. Curr Probl Diagn Radiol. 2011; 40: 95-115.

Rais-Bahrami K, Gilbert JC, Hartman GE, Chandra RS, Short BL. Right diaphragmatic eventration simulating a congenital diaphragmatic hernia. Am J Perinatol. 1996; 13: 241-3.

Harjai MM, Indrajit IK, Kansra M. Isolated dextrogastria simulating congenital diaphragmatic hernia: a diagnostic dilemma. Asian J Surg. 2010; 33: 59-62.

Aga P, Parashari UC, Parihar A, Singh R, Kohli N. MRI in isolated dextrogastria with eventration of the right hemidiaphragm with associated mesentero-axial volvulus. Pediatr Radiol. 2010; 40: 1576-8.

Nagdeve NG, Sarin YK. Volvulus complicating dextrogastria in an infant. Indian Pediatr. 2007; 44: 142-4.

Chang SW, Lee HC, Yeung CY, Chan WT, Hsu CH, Kao HA, Hung HY, Chang JH, Sheu JC, Wang NL. A twenty-year review of early and late-presenting congenital Bochdalek diaphragmatic hernia: are they different clinical spectra? Pediatr Neonatol. 2010; 51: 26-30.

Delport SD. Aftermath of failed diagnosis of late-presenting congenital diaphragmatic hernias. S Afr J Surg. 1996; 34: 69-72.

Numanoglu A, Steiner Z, Millar A, Cywes S. Delayed presentation of congenital diaphragmatic hernia. S Afr J Surg. 199; 35: 74-6.

Kitano Y, Lally KP, Lally PA. Congenital Diaphragmatic Hernia Study Group. Late-presenting congenital diaphragmatic hernia. J Pediatr Surg. 2005; 40:1839-43.

Elhalaby EA, Abo Sikeena MH. Delayed presentation of congenital diaphragmatic hernia. Pediatr Surg Int. 2002; 18: 480-5.

Zaleska-Dorobisz U, Bagłaj M, Sokołowska B, Ładogórska J, Moroń K. Late presenting diaphragmatic hernia: clinical and diagnostic aspects. Med Sci Monit. 2007; 13:137-46.

Cigdem MK, Onen A, Otcu S, Okur H. Late presentation of bochdalek-type congenital diaphragmatic hernia in children: a 23-year experience at a single center. Surg Today. 2007; 37: 642-5.

Pandey A, Tandon RK, Kureel SN, Wakhlu A, Rawat J. Evaluation of congenital diaphragmatic hernia in a tertiary health center of a developing country: management and survival. Hernia. 2008; 12:189-92.

Koziarkiewicz M, Piaseczna-Piotrowska A. Late manifestation of congenital diaphragmatic hernia - case report. Med Wieku Rozwoj. 2011; 15:106-9.

Marhuenda C, Guillén G, Sánchez B, Urbistondo A, Barceló C. Endoscopic repair of late-presenting Morgagni and Bochdalek hernia in children: case report and review of the literature. J Laparoendosc Adv Surg Tech A. 2009; 19: S95-101.

Al-Shehri MA, Al-Binali AM, Eid WA, Osinowo OA, Mohammed NE. Late presentation of a right Bochdalek hernia with a right intrathoracic stomach and organo-axial torsion. Saudi Med J. 2005l; 26:1122-6.

Pousios D, Panagiotopoulos N, Argyriou P, Piyis A. Diagnosis and surgical management of diaphragmatic agenesis in an adult: Report of a case. Surg Today. 2010; 40: 357-9.

Raut A, Jadhav S, Vora R, Mandke J, Sarode V, Kittur D. Right congenital diaphragmatic hernia associated with anorectal malformation. J Pediatr Surg. 2010; 45: E25-7.

Hussain N, Dawrant MJ, Firmin RK. A unique case of a congenital diaphragmatic hernia in a boy with albinism. J Pediatr Surg. 2009; 44: e21-2.

Palma G, Giordano R, Russolillo V, Vosa C. Cardiac defect with diaphragmatic hernia and left lung agenesis--heart disease and other anomalies. Thorac Cardiovasc Surg. 2010; 58: 439-40.

Kamath GS, Borkar S, Chauhan A, Chidanand B, Kashyap N, Warrier R. A rare case of congenital diaphragmatic hernia with ectopic liver and absent pericardium. Ann Thorac Surg. 2010; 89: 36-7.

Makis W, Rush C. Liver herniation through the foramen of Morgagni: a pitfall in oncologic F-18 FDG PET/CT evaluation of the anterior mediastinum. Clin Nucl Med. 2011; 36: 491-3.

Niramis R, Poocharoen W, Watanatittan S.Bilateral Morgagni hernias association with left Bochdalek diaphragmatic hernia: a very rare anomaly. J Med Assoc Thai. 2008; 91: S157-60.

5

Genetics of Congenital Diaphragmatic Hernia

Gabriele Starker, Ismini Staboulidou, Cornelia Beck,
Konstantin Miller and Constantin von Kaisenberg
Hannover Medical School
Germany

1. Introduction

The frequency of congenital diaphragmatic hernia in live borns is 1:3000 (Langham et al., 1996). Congenital diaphragmatic hernia is a potentially life threatening condition and is associated with significant perinatal mortality and morbidity (Skari et al., 2000; Torfs et al., 1992).

The most important prognostic parameter is the presence / absence of chromosomal abnormalities (Table 1) and / or genetic syndromes (Table 2), although factors such as pulmonary lung hypoplasia, a liver displaced into the thorax and associated anomalies may be similarly important (Fig. 1).

This chapter deals with the genetics of CDH looking both at numerical and structural chromosomal abnormalities and the known mutations and genetic syndromes. This has important implications for the diagnostic workup during pregnancy and the subsequent management of the pregnancy and birth.

2. Classification of congenital diaphragmatic hernia

In about 80-85% of CDH the hernia is on the left side, in 10-15% on the right side and in 5% bilaterally (Dott et al., 2003). Most diaphragmatic defects involve the posterior and lateral aspects of the diaphragm, such as the **posterolateral** or **Bochdalek** CDH (80-90%), often accompanied by herniation of the stomach, intestines, liver and spleen into the chest (Torfs et al., 1992). In cases of aplasia or agenesis of the diaphragm, CDH is summarized under the **large Bochdalek defects** (Baglaj et al., 1999). In about 5%, the defect is in other locations affecting e.g. the anterior retrosternal or parasternal diaphragm, referred to as the **Morgagni-Larrey** hernia. In these cases, there can be hernation of liver or intestines into the chest cavity. Other anterior hernias are associated with **Cantrell's Pentalogy** including defects of the supraumbilical midline abdominal wall, the lower sternum, the diaphragmatic pericardium and there may be ectopia cordis. Central hernias affect the tendinous portion of the diaphragm.

3. Etiology

Etiological concepts include abnormalities of the retinoic pathways, the mesenchymal development and the dual hit hypothesis.

The retinoic hypothesis: some of the loci such as 15q26, 8p23.1 and 8q23 are involved in the retinoic acid pathway and metabolism and are strongly association with CDH (Beurskens et al., 2010; Greer et al., 2003).

The mesenchymal-hit hypothesis: CDH originates from an abnormal development of the primordial pleuroperitoneal folds (PPF), important structures of the embryogenesis of the diaphragm. Genes affecting PPF development are COUP-TFII, FOG2, GATA-4, WT1 and Disp1, expressed in the non-muscular mesenchymal components of the diaphragm (Clugston et al., 2006; Clugston et al., 2008; Kantarci et al., 2010). Disp 1 is expressed in the primordial pleuroperitoneal fold (PPF), in diaphragmatic tissues and in the developing lung mesothelium, epithelium, and mesenchyme (Kantarci et al., 2010).

The dual-hit hypothesis: the lung is first hit by primary pulmonary underdevelopment through arrest of the alveolar development at the mid-canalicular stage, secondly the lung is hit by mechanical compression (Keijzer et al., 2000).

It has become increasingly evident that genetic factos play an important role in the etiology of CDH. There is one known mutation in a single gene causing isolated CDH. For complex CDH several single gene mutation in various genes have been identified responsible for a specific syndrome. Alternatively, complex CDH may be associated with rearrangement in specific gene loci. However, it is still uncertain whether genetic factors are the sole cause of CDH.

The evidence from teratogen and dietary-induced animal models is suggestive of differences in nutritional habits and other environmental factors contributing to a different susceptibility and phenotypical outcome (Beurskens et al., 2009).

4. Prognostic factors

The fate of the neonate will essentially be determined by an underlying systemic chromosomal or genetic abnormality on the one hand and by pulmonary hypoplasia or additional anatomical defects on the other hand. Anomalies may or may not be associated with chromosomal problems.

The total mortality in CDH is up to 50% and may be as little as 10-20% in isolated cases (Colvin et al., 2005; Skari et al., 2000; Stege et al., 2003). In the presence of associated anatomical defects as in complex CDH, the mortality rate is increased (Cohen et al., 2002). Other factors are the size of the diaphragmatic defect (Lally et al., 2007), the side with right-sided CDH showing a higher mortality than those on the left, presumably because the liver is up, and bilateral CDH showing the highest mortality (Skari et al., 2000). Other prognostic determinants are if the liver ís up in the chest or below the diaphragm (Albanese et al., 1998), the degree of pulmonary hypoplasia and the development and degree of pulmonary hypertension in the perinatal period (reviewed in (Pober et al., 1993)).

5. Isolated CDH

An isolated CDH is a defect, which may be associated with additional anomalies, but these affect fetal hemodynamics or describe mechanical consequences of the CDH. Those defects include dextroposition of the heart, a small compressed heart, tricuspid or mitral valve regurgitation, pulmonary hypoplasia, a patent foramen ovale or ductus arteriosus, malrotation or incomplete rotation of bowel, undescended testes and accessory spleen (Pober, 2008). The recurrence risk of isolated CDH in an sibling is 1-2% (Czeizel & Kovacs, 1985; Pober et al., 2005).

To date there is only one known de novo mutation in the FOG2 gene, which is the only single gene mutation causing isolated CDH (Ackerman et al., 2005).

6. Complex CDH

A complex CDH is a situation, where the CDH is associated with additional malformations. There may be associated chromosomal abnormalities, monogenetic syndromes or cases of complex CDH not part of a known genetic syndrome (Pober, 2008).

In about 60%, CDH is isolated, in 40% complex CDH due to the presence of additional major malformations, chromosomal abnormalities or single gene disorders (Colvin et al., 2005; Dott et al., 2003; Skari et al., 2000; Torfs et al., 1992).

6.1 CDH and chromosomal abnormalities

The following paragraph specifies the most common numerical and structural abnormalities including deletions, duplications and translocations associated with CDH. Since chromosomal abnormalities of nearly all chromosomes have been described in association with CDH we present "hot spots", which are likely to contain genes contributing to CDH and which are the best characterized to date. For a detailed list of chromosomal abnormalities we suggest excellent reviews which have been published (Holder et al., 2007; Lurie, 2003).

6.1.1 Numerical chromosomal abnormalities

Numerical chromosomal abnormalities are found in about 10% of CDH.

Congenital diaphragmatic hernia is part of the common chromosomal abnormalities such as the trisomies 18 (10%) and 13 (6%) and in triploidy (2%) (Table 1) (Snijders & Nicolaides, 1996). It has also been described in Turner syndrome (Bohn, 2002). The frequency of chromosomal abnormalities in the total CDH group is 18%, 2% if the CDH is isolated and 34%, if there are additional anomalies (Snijders & Nicolaides, 1996).

In a series of 155 cases of **Trisomy 21**, there is nuchal edema (38%), mild hydronephrosis (30%), short femur (28%), cardiac abnormalities (26%), abnormal hands and feet (25%), hydrops (20%), small for gestational age (20%), cerebral ventriculomegaly (16%), brachycephaly (15%), chorioid plexus cysts (8%), duodenal atresia (8%), enlarged cisterna magna (7%), absent stomach (3%), talipes (3%) and no case of CDH (Snijders & Nicolaides, 1996). In Trisomy 21, the frequency of CDH is low and of the Morgangi-type (Parmar et al., 2001).

In a series of 137 cases of **Trisomy 18**, there is intrauterine growth restriction (74%), there are abnormal hands and feet (72%), strawberry-shaped head (54%), micrognathia (53%), cardiac abnormalities (52%), chorioid plexus cysts (45%), exomphalos (31%), talipes (30%), brachycephaly (29%), short femur (25%), esophageal atresia or absent stomach (20%), mild hydronephrosis (16%), cerebral ventriculomegaly (14%), other renal abnormalities (12%), diaphragmatic hernia (10%), posteria fossa cyst (10%), facial cleft (10%) (Benacerraf et al., 1988; Snijders & Nicolaides, 1996; Tongsong et al., 2002).

In a series of 54 cases of **Trisomy 13,** there is intrauterine growth restriction (61%), abnormal hands and feet (52%), cardiac abnormalities (43%), facial cleft and holoprosencephaly (39%), mild hydronephrosis (37%), brachycephaly (26%), enlarged cisterna magna (25%), microcephaly (24%), other renal abnormalities (24%), nuchal edema (22%), exomphalos (17%), posterior fossa cyst (15%), talipes (11%), short femur (9%), cerebral ventriculomegaly (9%), micrognathia (9%), hydrops (7%), diaphragmatic hernia (6%) (Snijders & Nicolaides, 1996).

Fetal abnormality	Chromosomal defect				
	Trisomy			Triploidy	Turner
	21 n=155	18 n=137	13 n=54	n=50	n=65
Skull/Brain					
Strawberry shaped head	-	54%	-	-	-
Brachycephaly	15%	29%	26%	10%	32%
Microcephaly	-	1%	24%	-	5%
Ventriculomegaly	16%	14%	9%	18%	2%
Holoprosencephaly	-	3%	39%	-	-
Choroid plexus cysts	8%	47%	2%	-	-
Absent corpus callosum	-	7%	-	-	-
Posterior fossa cyst	1%	10%	15%	6%	-
Enlarged cisterna magna	7%	16%	25%	-	-
Face/Neck					
Facial cleft	1%	10%	39%	2%	-
Micrognathia	1%	53%	9%	44%	-
Nuchal oedema	38%	5%	22%	4%	6%
Cystic hygromata	1%	2%	-	-	88%
Chest					
Diaphragmatic hernia	-	10%	6%	2%	-
Cardiac abnormality	26%	52%	43%	16%	48%
Abdomen					
Exomphalos	-	31%	17%	2%	-
Duodenal atresia	8%	-	2%	-	-
Absent stomach	3%	20%	2%	2%	-
Mild hydronephrosis	30%	16%	37%	4%	8%
Other renal abnormalities	7%	12%	24%	6%	6%
Other					
Hydrops	20%	4%	7%	2%	80%
Small for gestational age	20%	74%	61%	100%	55%
Relatively short femur	28%	25%	9%	60%	59%
Abnormal hands / feet	25%	72%	52%	76%	2%
Talipes	3%	30%	11%	8%	-

Table 1. Incidence of ultrasound abnormalities in 461 fetuses with chromosomal defects that were examined at the Harris Birthright Research Centre for Fetal Medicine (Snijders & Nicolaides, 1996).

In a series of 65 cases of **Turner syndrome**, there was no case with diaphgragmatic hernia (Snijders & Nicolaides, 1996).

In a series of 50 cases of **Triploidy**, the main features were intrauterine growth restriction (100%), abnormal hands and feet (76%), short femur (60%), micrognathia (44%) and diaphragmatic hernia (2%) (Snijders & Nicolaides, 1996).

6.1.2 Supernumerary derivative chromosome 22 syndrome

+der(22)t(11;22)(q23;q11), Emanuel syndrome OMIM #609029

This syndrome is caused by a duplication of chromosomal segments of chromosomes 11 and 22 due to a 3:1 malsegregation of a common reciprocal translocation between the long arms of chromosome 11 and 22. In this partial duplication 11(q23-qter) and 22(pter-q11) complex CDH has been observed (Kadir et al., 1997). There is growth retardation, mental retardation, cardiovascular malformation, craniofacial anomalies (including preauricular tags or sinuses, micrognathia, ear anomalies, cleft or high-arched palate), microcephaly, kidney abnormalities and genital abnormalities in males (Carter et al., 2009).

6.1.3 Structural chromosomal abnormalities

In this section, we present examples for missing genes or genes with disturbed function caused by deletions or micro-deletions or by abnormal structure formation of chromosomes, clinically resulting in CDH.

Deletions

del(1)(q41-q42.12) OMIM #612530

This abnormality affects the DISP 1 gene (Kantarci et al., 2010; Shaffer et al., 2007). The clinical features are CDH and holoprosencephaly. There is a clinical overlap with the Fryns syndrome (Kantarci et al., 2006).

del(4)(p16) Wolf-Hirschhorn syndrome (WHS) OMIM #194190

This abnormality affects 4p16.3. The clinical features include pre- and postnatal growth deficiency, developmental disability of variable degree, characteristic craniofacial features ('greek warrior helmet' appearance of the high-arched eyebrows and the nose, high forehead, prominent glabella, hypertelorism, protruding eyes, epicanthal folds, short philtrum, distinct mouth with downturned corners, and micrognathia), seizures, closure defects (cleft lip or palate, coloboma of the eye) and cardiac septal defects. Diaphragmatic hernia is a rare feature of the WHS phenotype (Casaccia et al., 2006; Sergi et al., 1998).

del(8)(p23.1) OMIM #222400

This deletion removes GATA-4, a gene which is important for the development of the diaphragm and the heart and lung (Ackerman et al., 2007). Clinical features include cardiovascular malformations, intellectual disability, mild facial dysmorphology, renal anomalies and CDH in up to 20%.

del(8)(q23.1) OMIM #610187

This deletion removes the ZFPM2 (FOG 2) gene. The clinical result is isolated CDH and pulmonary hypoplasia (Ackerman et al., 2005; Bleyl et al., 2007).

del(15)(q26.1-q26.2) OMIM #142340

There may be a de novo deletion of terminal 15q or a loss of chromosomal material caused by unbalanced translocations or ring chromosome 15 formation (Pober et al., 2005). The 15q26.1-q26.2 deletion may result in removal of COUP-TFII, CDH2, RGMA, SIAT8B and MEF2A (Biggio et al., 2004; Klaassens et al., 2005). Epigenetic factors likely contribute to the development of CDH for this gene. The clinical phenotype is intrauterine growth retardation, intellectual disability, facial dysmorphology, limb, renal and cardiovascular malformations, hypoplastic genitalia and CDH. There is a high mortality of 30-60% in newborns (Klaassens et al., 2007; Langham et al., 1996).

Isochromosome

Isochromosome 12p (Tetrasomy 12p) Pallister-Killian syndrome (PKS) OMIM #601803

This syndrome is characerized by the mosaic presence of a supernumerary isochromosome of the short arm of chromosome 12 in some tissues. This results in 4 copies of the genes on chromosome 12p (Struthers et al., 1999). The clinical features include (prenatally): short limbs, CNS anomalies, cerebral ventricular dilatation, craniofacial dysmorphology, excess fluid accumulation such as nuchal edema/hydrops fetalis, polyhydramnion and CDH in 10-50% (Doray et al., 2002; Mowery-Rushton et al., 1997). In addition postnatally there is bitemporal sparseness of hair, facial dysmorphology (brachycephaly, high broad forehead, ocular hypertelorism, low-set ears, broad nasal bridge, anteverted nostrils, long philtrum), short neck with nuchal skin redundancy, short broad hands, syndactyly, linear streaks of skin hyperpigmentation, normal growth, seizures and moderate intellectual disability.

There is some clinical overlap with Fryns Syndrome. A large number of fetuses are stillborn or die in the neonatal period.

Tetrasomy 12 mosaicism can be diagnosed from skin fibroblasts, chorionic villi and amniotic fluid cells, whereas in lymphocytes from cordocentesis, the isochromosome is likely to be missed (Doray et al., 2002).

6.2 Monogenic syndromes with CDH as common symptom

There are more than 70 syndromes in which diaphragmatic hernia has been observed (Slavotinek, 2007). This paragraph deals with selected syndromes most commonly associated with CDH. For further syndromes in which CDH has been described only in a few cases see Online Mendelian Inheritance In Man (OMIM) of John Hopkins University.

Defects on almost all chromosomes have been described in patients with CDH which considerably complicates the unravelling of the etiology of CDH (Holder et al., 2007). The genetic heterogeneity might reflect interactions of several candidate genes at the protein level. Certain proteins function at different steps of a pathway and errors may therefore occur at many levels, causing different specific disease phenotypes (Klaassens et al., 2009).

Cornelia de Lange syndrome 1 (CDLS1) OMIM #122470

CDLS is in about 50-60% a de novo autosomal dominant mutation in the NIPBL gene on 5p13.1. (Gillis et al., 2004), there are also in about 5% X-linked mutations in the SMC1A gene on Xp11.2, a mild variant of CDLS is caused by a mutation in the SMC3 gene on 10q25.2.

The prevalence is 0.6-10:100.000 individuals.

Clinical features include (prenatally): intrauterine growth restriction, hypoplastic forearms, underdevelopment of the hands, typical facial defects and diaphragmatic hernia (Manouvrier et al., 1996). Postnatally, growth retardation, hirsutism, mental retardation, microcephaly, upper limb reduction defects such as oligodactyly, dysmorphic facial appearance (low anterior hairline, synophrys, arched eyebrowns, long eyelashes, small upturned nose with a long philtrum, thin upper lip, downturned corners of the mouth, small widely spaced teeth) are found (Gillis et al., 2004), in 5-10% with CDH (Martinez-Frias et al., 1998). There is reduced survival. The phenotype is highly variable. The empiric risk for a sib of an affected child is between 2 and 5%.

Prenatal molecular genetic testing is available.

Craniofrontonasal syndrome (CFNS) OMIM #304110

CFNS is a mutations in the EFNB1 gene on Xq12 (Wieland et al., 2004). Craniofrontonasal syndrome is an X-linked developmental disorder that shows paradoxically greater severity in heterozygous females than in hemizygous males. A possible explanation could be, that EFNB1 escapes X inactivation. There is some overlap with Hypertelorism of the Teebi Type (OMIM #145420) which includes CDH.

The prevalence is unknown.

Clinical features include in **Females:** coronal craniosynostosis, craniofacial dysmorphism: hypertelorism, broad nasal bridge, broad nasal tip, facial asymmetry, frontal bossing, widow's peak, curly hair, cleft lip and palate, a variety of skeletal abnormalities such as grooved nails and CDH.

Clinical features include in **Males:** hypertelorism or telecanthus, short stature, potentially mild musculoskeletal abnormalities (Saavedra et al., 1996; Vasudevan et al., 2006).

Prenatal molecular genetic testing is available.

Donnai-Barrow syndrome (facio-oculo-acoustico-renal syndrome) OMIM #222448

This is a mutation in the LPR2 gene on 2q23.3-2q31.1, inheritance is autosomal recessive (Chassaing et al., 2003; Gripp et al., 1997; Kantarci et al., 2007).

The prevalence is unknown.

Clinical features include high myopia, coloboma, hypertelorism, complete or partial agenesis of the corpus callosum, sensorineural hearing loss, cardiac defects, facial dysmorphology (wide anterior fontanelle, downslanting palpebral fissures, epicanthal folds, short nose with a broad tip, low-set posteriorly angulated ears), developmental delay, low-molecular-weight proteinuria, omphalocele and in about 50% CDH (Donnai & Barrow, 1993).

Prenatal molecular genetic testing at present is available only for research.

Fryns syndrome OMIM #229850

The clinical phenotype of Fryns syndrome has been observed in association with mosaicism for a tandem duplication of 1q24-q31.2 (Clark & Fenner-Gonzales, 1989), but also in association with anomalies of chromosome 6, 15 and 22 respectively (de Jong et al., 1989; Dean et al., 1991;

Krassikoff & Sekhon, 1990) indicating genetic heterogeneity of the syndrome. Thus, these cases may all represent mimics of the mendelian syndrome and have no significance as to the location of the gene for the recessive disorder. The gene responsible for Fryns syndrome is not yet known. There is an autosomal recessive Fryns (OMIM #229850), there is a type with chromosomal microdeletion and microduplication phenocopies and there are autosomal recessive phenocopies due to mutations in other genes (Pober, 2008).

The prevalence is 7:100.000 live births (Ayme et al., 1989).

A common finding in complex CDH, in about 10%, is Fryns syndrome (Slavotinek, 2004), therefore it is the most likely diagnosis in the clinical finding of CDH with associated anomalies (Fryns et al., 1979; Neville et al., 2002).

Guidelines for classifying Fryns syndrome using 5 categories (Lin et al., 2005):

- CDH: approximately 80% have a congenital abnormality of the diaphragm, most commonly Bochdalek's hernia.
- pulmonary hypoplasia: always accompanies CDH.
- facial dysmorphology: coarsened face, flattened nasal bridge, thickened nasal tip, long philtrum, hypertelorism, non-specific ear anomalies, widely spaced eyes, macrostomia, micrognathia.
- distal digital hypoplasia: small nails and/or distal phalanges.
- characteristic pattern of additional anomalies: mainly cardiovascular, renal and brain malformations, at least one of: polyhydramnios, cloudy cornea and/or microphthalmia, orofacial cleft, brain malformation, cardiovascular malformation, renal dysplasia and cortical renal cysts, gastrointestinal malformations, genital malformations.
- similarly affected sibling.

A classical definition of Fryns syndrome includes four of the six clinical findings, a more widely definition three out of six features.

Key ultrasound features include polyhydramnios in half of the cases, CDH and cystic hygroma (Manouvrier-Hanu et al., 1996). The prognosis is poor as there are only about 15% survivors in the neonatal period and severe mental retardation is common in survivors (Slavotinek, 2004).

Matthew-Wood syndrome (PDAC or PMD syndrome) OMIM #601186

This syndrome is caused by mutations in STRA6 on 15q24.1, a membrane receptor for vitamin A retinol binding protein and is autosomally recessive inherited (Pasutto et al., 2007).

Only a few cases have been reported so far, therefore the prevalence cannot be estimated to date.

Clinical features include microphthalmia or anophthalmia, pulmonary hypoplasia or agenesis, cardiac defects and CDH in up tp 50% (Chitayat et al., 2007). The prognosis is poor as there is early lethality in most cases.

Prenatal molecular genetic testing at present is available only for research.

Spondylocostal dysostosis 1 SCD1 (Jarcho-Levin syndrome) OMIM #277300

This syndrome is most frequently caused by a mutation in DLL3 on 19q13 and is autosomally recessive inherited. There are further autosomally recessive types of spondylocostal dysostosis

(SCD2-4) and the respective gene mutations are: MESP2 on 15q26.1 (without CDH) OMIM #608681, LFNG on 7p22.4 (without CDH) OMIM #609813, HES7 on 17p13.1 (without CDH) OMIM #613686 and SCD 5, autosomally dominant, OMIM #122600.

The prevalence is unknown.

Clinical featues include multiple contiguous vertebral abnormalities, malalignment of the ribs with variable points of intercostal fusion, and often a reduction in rib number, shortened trunk, short neck, hemivertebrae, vertebral fusion, scoliosis, severe expression with respiratory compromise and death resulting from a significant reduction in chest size, cleft palate, renal anomalies, patent ductus arteriosus and CDH (Day & Fryer, 2003; Rodriguez et al., 2004).

Spondylothoracic dysplasia (STD) OMIM #277300

This syndrome shares phenotypic similarities with spondylocostal dysostosis. Main features are a "fan-like" configuration of the chest in which the ribs appear to emanate from only a few vertebral bodies, additional cardinal abnormalities include malformed vertebrae and ribs, genitourinary abnormalities and hernias and CDH (Day & Fryer, 2003; Shehata et al., 2000).

Molecular genetic testing is available for DLL3, MESP2, LFNG (HES7 research only).

Simon-Golabi-Behmel syndrome type 1 OMIM #312870

This is a syndrome caused by a mutation in the GPC3 gene on Xp26.2 (Pilia et al., 1996). It is X-linked recessive inherited.

The prevalence is unknown.

Clinical features include prenatal or postnatal overgrowth, coarse facial features with hypertelorism, macrosomia, abdominal wall defects (including umbilical hernia and omphalocele), skeletal anomalies (including brachydactyly, postaxial polydactyly, cutaneous syndactyly), renal anomalies (hydronephrosis, cystic dysplatic kidney), supernumerary nipples, (Neri et al., 1998; Sakazume et al., 2007), an increased risk of embryonal tumors such as Wilms tumor and hepatocellular carcinoma (Li et al., 2001). The overgrowth is present from the prenatal period accompanied by macroglossia, an advanced bone age, organomegaly and neonatal hypoglycaemia (Neri et al., 1998). Structural and conductive cardiac abnormalities are seen in 35%, there is also congenital hypotonia, seizures, brain malformations and developmental disability. The prognosis is poor as approximately 50% die in the neonatal period, survivors have low-normal intelligence.

Molecular genetic testing is available.

WT1-opathies

Denys-Drash syndrome OMIM #194080, **Frasier syndrome** OMIM #136680, **Meacham syndrome** OMIM #608978 and **WAGR syndrome** OMIM #194072

This group of genetic syndromes is caused by a mutation in WT1 on 11p13 and is autosomal dominant.

The WT1 gene is expressed in the septum transversum of the diaphragm and in the pleural and abdominal mesothelial tissue that form the diaphragm (Moore et al., 1998). Pathological studies have demonstrated defects in the formation of the primordial pleuroperitoneal folds (PPF) in WT1 null mice (Clugston et al., 2006).

It is likely that heterozygous mutations/deletions of WT1 increase the likelihood that an individual will develop CDH. Environmental factors and differences in genetic background may also play a role in determining whether an individual with a WT1 abnormality develops CDH (Scott et al., 2005). Although WT1 may play an important role in diaphragm development, abnormalities in WT1 do not appear to be a common cause of isolated diaphragmatic hernia.

Common features are CDH (not 100%), genital abnormalities and associated anomalies (Antonius et al., 2008; Cho et al., 2006; Devriendt et al., 1995; Killeen et al., 2002; Scott et al., 2005; Suri et al., 2007).

The prevalence of these rare diseases are unknown.

Denys-Drash syndrome OMIM #194080 triad consisting of nephropathy, Wilms tumor, and genital abnormalities (male pseudohermaphroditism) (Cho et al., 2006; Devriendt et al., 1995). Death is usually due to renal failure by average age 3, most cases are sporadic.

Frasier syndrome OMIM #136680 46,XY males with normal female external genitalia, hypospadias, cryptorchidism, streak gonads, progressive nephrotic syndrome with proteinuria secondary to focal and segmental glomerular sclerosis and gonadoblastoma (Denamur et al., 2000).

Meacham syndrome OMIM #608978 complex cardiovascular malformations, lung defects including severe pulmonary hypoplasia, congenital bronchiectasis, pulmonary sequestration, ambigouous external genitalia or undervirilized male external genitalia with duplication of the vagina in chromosomal males (Meacham et al., 1991; Suri et al., 2007).

WAGR syndrome OMIM #194072 Wilms tumor (50%), aniridia, genitourinary anomalies, mental retardation, CDH is rare, genes are WT1 and PAX6 (Scott et al., 2005).

Molecular genetic testing is available.

6.3 Selected syndromes with CDH as an occasional finding

Apert syndrome OMIM #101200

This syndrome is caused be a mutation in the FGFR2 gene on 10q26.13, autosomally dominant.

The estimated frequency of Apert syndrome is 1 in 160.000 births.

Clinical features include craniosynostosis, mid-face hypoplasia, ocular hypertelorism, fusion of cervical vertebrae, varying degree of bilateral soft tissue and bony syndactyly of hands and feet and developmental delay/intellectual disability in approximately 50% (Pober et al., 1993).

Molecular genetic testing is available.

Beckwith-Wiedemann syndrome OMIM #130650

This syndrome is caused by dysregulation of imprinted genes within the chromosome 11p15.5 region including CDKN1C, H19, and LIT1. Mutations in the NSD1 gene on chromosome 5q35 have been identified in two cases. It can be transmitted autosomal dominant while the majority of cases are a single occurrence in the family.

The population incidence is estimated to be 1:13.700 births. This figure is likely an underestimate as milder phenotypes may not be ascertained. The incidence is equal in males and females with the notable exception of monozygotic twins that show a dramatic excess of females (Weksberg et al., 2010).

Clinical features are overgrowth during the latter half of pregnancy and in the first few years of life while adult heights are generally in the normal range. Fetal adrenocortical cytomegaly is a pathognomonic finding during prenatal ultrasound examination. Additional features involve abdominal wall defects, earlobe creases or pits behind the upper ear, macroglossia and visceromegaly involving liver, spleen, pancreas, kidneys, or adrenals. Renal anomalies may include primary malformations, renal medullary dysplasia, nephrocalcinosis, and nephrolithiasis. Hypoglycemia is reported in 30 to 50% of babies and there is a predisposition to embryonal malignancies, with Wilms tumor and hepatoblastoma being the most common. CDH is a rare phenotypic finding (Pober et al., 1993; Turleau et al., 1984; Weksberg et al., 2010).

Molecular genetic testing is available.

CHARGE syndrome OMIM #214800

Most cases result from de novo mutation in the CHD7 gene on 8q12.1 or in the SEMA3E gene on 7q21.11. The inheritance is autosomal dominant.

The incidence is 1:12.000 births.

The syndrome presents clinically with coloboma of the eye, cardiovascular malformations, choanal atresia or stenosis, growth and mental retardation, genital anomalies, ear anomalies, hearing loss and microcephaly (Casaccia et al., 2008; Vissers et al., 2004).

Molecular genetic testing is available.

Trigonocephaly OMIM #211750

This syndrome is caused by a mutation in the CD96 gene on 3q13.1-q13.2. The inheritance is autosomal recessive.

The estimated incidence is 1:12.000 births.

The clinical presentation includes metopic craniosynostosis, orofacial anomalies (deep midline palatal groove, broad alveolar ridges, and multiple frenula), genital anomalies, cardiovascular defects, short limbs, polydactyly, loose skin and intellectual disability (Addor et al., 1995)

Molecular genetic testing is not available.

Coffin-Siris syndrome OMIM #135900

This syndrome is caused by a mutation in the 7q32-q34 region. The specific gene and the inheritance are not yet known as the majority of cases are sporadic. Affected sibs have been described. Only about 40 cases are published and the prevalence is estimated to be less than 1:1.000.000. The most likely mode of inheritance is autosomal recessive and the recurrence risk is 25% for sibs of an index case.

Clinical features are hypoplasia or absence of nail/phalanx of the fifth digit, scalp hypotrichosis, body hypertrichosis, facial dysmorphology (coarse face, wide mouth, full lips), growth retardation and intellectual disability. The female to male ratio is about 4:1 (Coffin & Siris, 1970; Haspeslagh et al., 1984).

Molecular testing is not available.

Cutis laxa, autosomal recessive type I OMIM #219100

This syndrome is caused by homozygosity for a missense mutation in the EFEMP2 gene, also known as FBLN4, on 11q13.1. There has also been described a mutation in the FBLN5 gene on 14q32.12 but this mutations has not been associated with CDH.

The prevalence of this syndrome has been estimated about 1-9:1.000.000.

The main clinical feature is soft, velvety, and transparent skin. Additional observations include hypotonia, emphysema, generalized arterial tortuosity, joint laxity, pectus excavatum and inguinal and diaphragmatic hernia (Hoyer et al., 2009; Hucthagowder et al., 2006). Oligohydramnios is a typical finding of prenatal ultrasound examination.

Molecular genetic testing is available.

Czeizel-Losonci syndrome OMIM #183802

The genetic cause of this syndrome is not yet known. It is autosomally dominant inherited. Molecular testing is not available. The incidence is not yet known as there are only a few cases described to date.

Clinical features are limb anomalies such as split hands/split feet, preaxial deficiency, and syndactyly, urinary tract obstruction, neural tube defects such as spina bifida and CDH (Czeizel & Losonci, 1987).

Ehlers Danlos syndrome type 1 OMIM #130000

This syndrome can be caused by a mutation in the collagen alpha-1(V) gene (COL5A1) on chromosome 9q34 or the collagen alpha-2(V) gene (COL5A2) on chromosome 2q31. One patient with EDS I has been reported to have a mutation in the collagen alpha-1(I) gene (COL1A1) on chromosome 17q. The inheritance is autosomal dominant.

Ehlers-Danlos syndrome (EDS) affects approximately 1:5.000 live births.

The main features of classic Ehlers-Danlos syndrome (EDS I and EDS II) are loose-jointedness and fragile, bruisable skin that heals with peculiar 'cigarette-paper' scars (Beighton et al., 1998; Zalis & Roberts, 1967). CDH is a rare feature.

Molecular genetic testing is available

Gershoni-Baruch syndrome OMIM 609545

The genetic cause of this syndrome is not yet known. It is autosomally recessive inherited (Franceschini et al., 2003). Molecular testing is not available. The incidence is not yet known as there are only a few cases described to date.

Clinical features include omphalocele, cardiovascular malformations, absent radial ray, vertebral anomalies, neural tube defect and a single umbilical artery (Gershoni-Baruch et al.,

1990). The perinatal lethality is very high. The clinical presentation of this syndrome overlaps with the DK phocomelia syndrome OMIM #223340 which also includes CDH.

Goltz syndrome (focal dermal hypoplasia) OMIM #305600

This syndrome is caused by a mutation in the PORCN gene on Xp11.23. The inheritance is X-linked dominant with a high in utero lethality in males. The majority of cases (95%) are sporadic. Ninety percent of cases are female. The frequency in a general population has not been estimated.

Goltz syndrome presents clinically with an asymmetric face, trunk and extremities, skin atrophy, subcutaneous nodules secondary of fat herniations through atrophic areas, alternating areas of hyper- and hypopigmentation, multiple mucous and perioral papilloma, oral anomalies including hypoplasia or aplasia of the teeth, enamel defects and malocclusion, ocular anomalies such as coloboma, microphthalmia and iris defects, osteopathia striata, skeletal abnormalities involving the extremities, short stature and mild mental deficiency. CDH is a rare feature (Han et al., 2000).

Molecular genetic testing is available

Hemifacial microsomia (Goldenhar syndrome) OMIM #164210

This syndrome is caused by mutation in the 14q32 region. Most cases are sporadic, but there are rare familial cases that exhibit autosomal dominant inheritance.(Pober et al., 1993; Rollnick & Kaye, 1983). Molecular testing is not available.

The estimated frequence is 1:3000-5000.

The malformations are caused by an abnormal morphogenesis of the first and second branchial arches and are often presented unilateral. Clinical features are facial asymmetry and ear anomalies. In addition to craniofacial anomalies, there may be cardiac, vertebral, and central nervous system defects (Pober et al., 1993). There is a slight male predominance (3:2).

Kabuki syndrome OMIM #147920

This syndrome is caused by mutation in the MLL2 gene on 12q12-q14, autosomally dominant inherited.

Kabuki syndrome is estimated to occur in at least 1:32.000 Japanese individuals.

Kabuki syndrome is a congenital mental retardation syndrome with additional features, including postnatal dwarfism, a peculiar facies characterized by long palpebral fissures with eversion of the lateral third of the lower eyelids, a broad and depressed nasal tip, large prominent earlobes, a cleft or high-arched palate, scoliosis, short fifth finger, persistence of fingerpads, radiographic abnormalities of the vertebrae, hands, and hip joints, and recurrent otitis media in infancy as well as cardiovascular malformations (Donadio et al., 2000; Genevieve et al., 2004; Niikawa et al., 1981)

Molecular genetic testing is available

Marfan syndrome OMIM #154700

This syndrome is caused by mutation in the FBN1 gene on 15q21.1 and is inherited autosomally dominant. However, about 25% of cases are due to new mutations.

The estimated prevalence of Marfan syndrome is between 1:5.000-10.000.

Marfan syndrome is caused by connective tissue dysplasia characterized by tall statue, disproportionately long extremities, subluxation of the lens, myopia, dilatation of the descending aorta, variety of other anomalies such as pectus deformities, kyphoscoliosis, joint hypermobility and dural ectasia, diaphragmatic abnormalities are rare (Revencu et al., 2004).

Molecular genetic testing is available

Mathieu syndrome there is no OMIM entry

The genetic cause of this syndrome has not been identified yet and therefore there is no molecular genetic testing available. Autosomal dominant inheritance is assumed.

The prevalence has not been described as there are only a few cases known.

Clinical features include facial dysmorphology such as epicanthal folds, short nose, depressed nasal bridge and micrognathia, cleft palate, short statue, short neck, vertebral abnormalities, tracheal abomalies and mild intellectual disability (Mathieu et al., 1993; Zelante & Ruscitto, 2003).

Microphthalmia with linear skin defect (MLS), MIDAS (MIcrophthalmia, Dermal Aplasia, Sclerocornea) **syndrome** OMIM #309801

This syndrome is caused by mutation in the HCCS gene on Xp22.2. There is X-linked dominant inheritance with in utero lethality for males.

It has been reported in less than 50 patients and the prevalence is estimated < 1:1.000.000.

The main clinical features in affected females are unilateral or bilateral microphthalmia and linear skin defects which are limited to the face and neck, consisting of areas of aplastic skin that heal with age to form hyperpigmented areas. Additional findings include sclerocornea, occasional cardiovascular malformations and genital anomalies (Wimplinger et al., 2006).

Molecular genetic testing is available.

Multiple pterygium syndrome, Escobar variant (non-lethal type) OMIM #265000

This syndrome is caused by a mutation in the CHRNG gene on 2q37.1. The inheritance is autosomal recessive (Entezami et al., 1998; Morgan et al., 2006). The prevalence of this syndrome has not been described.

Multiple pterygium syndromes comprise a group of multiple congenital anomaly disorders characterized by webbing (pterygia) of the neck, elbows, and/or knees and joint contractures (arthrogryposis). Other features can be skeletal defects and genital anomalies (Morgan et al., 2006).

Molecular genetic testing is available.

Myotubular myopathy 1 (MTM1) OMIM #310400

This syndrome is caused by a mutation in the MTM1 gene on Xq28. The inheritance is X-linked recessive (Laporte et al., 1996).

The incidence is estimated to be 1:50.000 newborn males.

This syndrome affects the skeletal muscle causing generalized muscle weakness. Other findings include it is congenital eventration of the diaphragm accompanied by diaphragmatic dysfunction causing serious respiratory problems (Grogan et al., 2005; Moerman et al., 1987). Therefore this syndrome is usually fatal in infancy. Some carrier females may manifest mild symptoms.

Molecular genetic testing is available.

Opitz GBBB syndrome type 1 OMIM #300000

This syndrome is caused by mutation in the MID1 gene on Xp22.2. The inheritance has been described as X-linked.

The prevalence has been estimated to be 1-9:100.000.

Clinical features include hypertelorism, hypospadias, cleft lip/palate, laryngotracheoesophageal abnormalities, imperforate anus, developmental delay, and cardiac defects. CDH is a rare feature (Enns et al., 1998).

Molecular genetic testing is available.

PAGOD syndrome OMIM 202660

The gene mutation causing this syndrome is not known but it has been hypothized to cause a defect on the vitamin A pathway.

Only about 6 cases have been described thus the prevalence and inheritance cannot be predicted.

Diagnostic criteria are pulmonary hypoplasia, cardiovascular malformations including hypoplasia of the pulmonary artery, hypo- or agonadism, ambiguous genitalia, omphalocele, dextrocardia and CDH (Kennerknecht et al., 1993).

Molecular testing is not available.

Pentalogy of Cantrell OMIM #313850 (included in THAS)

This extremely rare syndrome occurs sporadic and the genetic background has not been identified yet.

An evaluation of the prevalence of the pentalogy of Cantrell in the general population provided an estimate of 5.5:1.000.000 live births.

Diagnostic criteria are deficiency of anterior diaphragm, defect of the diaphragmatic pericardium, ectopia cordis or other cardiovascular malformations, supraumbilical abdominal wall defect and defect of lower sternum (Ghidini et al., 1988; Toyama, 1972). By definition, CDH is a part of this syndrome, but patients with incomplete pentalogy of Cantrell and without diaphragmatic hernias have been described (Song & McLeary, 2000). The survival is severely compromised because of the cardiac defects (Bittmann et al., 2004).

Molecular testing is not available.

Perlman syndrome OMIM #267000

The gene causing this syndrome is not known but autosomal recessive inheritance is suggested.

So far, about 30 patients have been reported in the literature, therefore the prevalence cannot be predicted yet.

Prenatal findings in ultrasound examination include fetal ascites without hydrops and polyhydramnios. Clinical manifestations are macrosomia, nephromegaly with renal hamartomas and most often nephroblastomatosis, hepatomegaly, hyperplasia of the endocrine pancreas accompanied by hyperinsulinism, typical facial appearance, and an increased risk for Wilms tumor. There is a high neonatal lethality with intellectual disability in survivors (Greenberg et al., 1988; Perlman, 1986).

Molecular testing is not available.

Poland syndrome OMIM #173800

This syndrome occurs sporadic and the genetic background has not been identified yet.

The prevalence at birth is about 1-3:100.000.

The clinical picture consists of unilateral absence or hypoplasia of the pectoralis muscle, most frequently involving the sternocostal portion of the pectoralis major muscle, and a variable degree of ipsilateral hand and digit anomalies, including symbrachydactyly (Hou & Wang, 1999; McGillivray & Lowry, 1977) .

Molecular testing is not available.

Swyer syndrome 46,XY sex reversal 1 OMIM #400044

About 30% of cases affected by this syndrome are caused by mutation or deletion of SRY on Yp11.31. The disorder is caused not only by mutations in the SRY gene, but by genes on the autosome and the X chromosome. There has been found no SRY mutations in persons with Swyer syndrome and CDH.

The prevalence is unknown.

Affected patients have a partial or complete gonadal dysgenesis. Individuals with 46,XY complete gonadal dysgenesis are phenotypically female; however, they do not develop secondary sexual characteristics at puberty and do not menstruate. They have bilateral 'streak gonads,' which typically consist of fibrous tissue and variable amounts of wavy ovarian stroma. A uterus and fallopian tube are present and external genitalia are female (Berkovitz et al., 1991; Kent et al., 2004).

Molecular genetic testing is available

Thoracoabdominal syndrome (THAS) OMIM #313850

This syndrome is caused by mutations in the Xq25-q26.1 region, the affected gene is unknown. The inheritance is presumably X-linked dominant.

The prevalence is estimated to be 1-9: 1.000.000.

Clinical features include adominal wall defects such as absent or hypoplastic abdominis rectus muscle, diaphragm defects, hypoplastic lung, occasional cardiovascular malformations and cleft palate (Carmi et al., 1990). This syndrome includes the malformations of the Pentalogy of Cantrell syndrome.

Molecular testing is not available.

6.4 CDH and other congenital malformations not part of a known genetic syndrome

In this section, we describe cases of CDH associated with additional anomalies, which do not constitute a specific genetic syndrome. The most common associated defects are cardiovascular, central nervous and of the musculoskeletal system.

CDH and cardiovascular malformations: these are found in about 10-15% of non-syndromic CDH cases (Dillon et al., 2000; Lin et al., 2007; Robert et al., 1997). A ventricular septal defect (VSD) or atrial septal defect (ASD) is the most frequent cardiac defect.

CDH and central nervous system abnormalities: they are found in about 5-10% of the non-syndromic CDH cases, particularly neural tube defects and hydrocephalus are common (Dillon et al., 2000; Dott et al., 2003).

CDH and limb abnormalities: in 10% of the non-syndromic CDH cases, syndactyly, polydactyly or limb reduction defects are found (Colvin et al., 2005; Stege et al., 2003; van Dooren et al., 2003).

CDH and genitourinary abnormalities: undescended testes commonly coexist with CDH, rarer findings are ectopic or absent testes and ectopic (thoracic) kidney. (Masturzo et al., 2001; Panda et al., 2009; van Dooren et al., 2003)

CDH and eye abnormalities: microphthalmia and anophthalmia are reported in several syndromes listed above (Macayran et al., 2002; Steiner et al., 2002).

6.5 CDH in multiple gestation

There is only little known about CDH in multigestational pregnancies. Of all cases with CDH about 3% occur in multiple gestation pregnancies (Pober et al., 2005; Robert et al., 1997). There are no published concordance ratios between MZ and DZ twins for CDH. Findings in the literature show that the majority of monozygotic twin pairs described in case reports or as part of a small series are concordant for CDH (Abe et al., 2001; Chao et al., 1997; Eichelberger et al., 1980; Gallot et al., 2003; Gencik et al., 1982; Gibbs et al., 1997; Lucas Talan et al., 1998; Machado et al., ; Mishalany & Gordo, 1986; Watanatittan, 1983). In contrast, most twin pairs reported as part of a consecutive series are discordant (David & Illingworth, 1976; Jancelewicz et al., 2010; Pober et al., 2005; Robert et al., 1997; Tonks et al., 2004; Torfs et al., 1992). Pober and coworkes (Pober et al., 2005) hypothesized that there is overreporting of concordantly affected twins in case reports and that CDH, even though it can be present in both members of a monozygous twin pair, it more frequently affects only one.

The reason for low sibling recurrence (less than 1%) and low monozygotic twin concordance of CDH can be due to different mechanisms, genetic and non-genetic. Genetic factors include incomplete penetrance, de novo chromosome abnormalities and new dominant mutations (Pober et al., 2005). It has been hypothesized that some cases of CDH may be due to mutations that interfere with normal epigenetic modifications (Austin-Ward & Taucher, 1999). Post-zygotic de novo mutations, as well as epigenetic differences are mechanisms proven to underly monozygotic twin discordance (Kondo et al., 2002; Weksberg et al., 2002).

Recently data about the outcome of multigestational pregnancies affected by CDH have been published (Jancelewicz et al., 2010). Jancelewicz and co-workes demonstrated that the live-born mortality for multigestational infants with CDH (20-30%) was roughly the same as for the general CDH population (25%). The incidence of adverse outcomes was high for both multiple and singleton pregnancies and seems to depend more on the severity of the CDH than the presence of multiple gestations. The gestational age at birth for multigestational pregnancies was found to be significantly lower than for the entire CDH cohort. However, prematurity is a concern in multigestational pregnancies in general accompanied by a higher morbidity and mortality for those infants. There seems to be no increases risk for the unaffected sibling in multigestational CDH pregnancies.

In summary, the outcome of multigestational pregnancies affected by CDH appear to be similar to those of singleton CDH pregnancies and the risk for morbidity and mortality likely depends more on CDH severity than the presence of multiple fetuses (Jancelewicz et al., 2010).

An example of a case of spontaneously conceived dichorionic diamniotic twin pregnancy discordant for CDH is presented here. The heart is on the right, there is mediastinal shift, the bowel is up in the thorax and there is a small right sided lung. The lung-to-head ratio is 2.1, which has a good prognosis (Fig. 1). The other fetus is structurally normal.

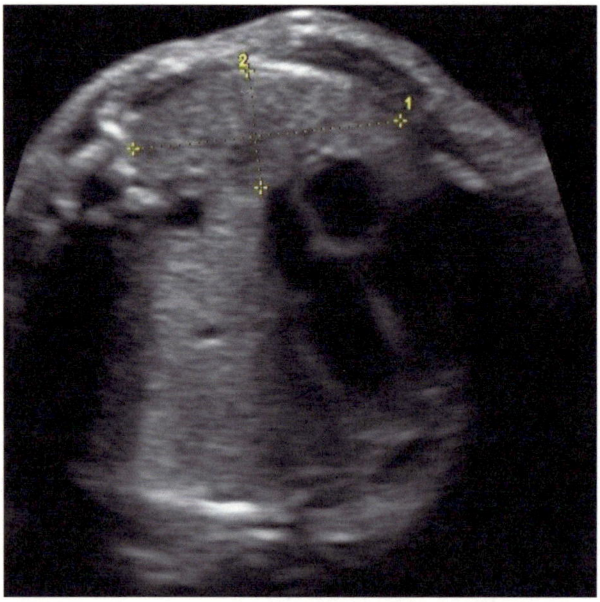

Fig. 1. CDH in a spontaneously conceived dichorionic diamniotic twin pregnancy discordant for diaphragmatic hernia at 32 weeks gestation.

Syndrome	OMIM	Clinic	Gene	Locus	Inheritance	Molecular testing	Prevalence
Cornelia de Lange syndrome 1	122470	low posterior hairline, anteverted nostrils, micrognathia, long philtrum, IUGR, limb abnormalities, 5-10% CDH	NIPBL	5p13.1	AD	+	0.6–10 : 100.000
Craniofrontalnasal syndrome	304110	craniofrontonasal dysostosis, hypertelorism, bifid nasal tip, musculoskeletal abnormalities, CDH is rare	EFNB1	Xq12	XL	+	Nk
Donnai-Barrow-Syndrome	222448	exomphalos, corpus callosum agenesis, hypertelorism, myopia, CDH, sensorineural deafness, 50-70% CDH	LPR2	2q23.3-2q31.1	AR	R	< 1 : 1.000.000
Fryns syndrome	229850	facial dysmorphology, distal digital hypoplasia, cardiovascular, renal and brain malformations, pulmonary hypoplasia, CDH up tp 80%	Nk	Nk	AR	-	7 : 100.000
Matthew-Wood syndrome	601186	microphthalmia / anophthalmia, pulmonary hypoplasia / agenesis, cardiac defects, CDH - 50%	STRA6	15q24.1	AR	R	Nk
Spondylocostal dysostosis 1	277300	short statue, hemivertebrae, fused vertebrae, rib anomalies, CDH is rare	DLL3	19q13	AR	+	Nk
Simpson-Golabi-Behmel syndrome	312870	kephalic and facial anomalies: makrokephaly, hypertelorism, broad flat nasal bridge, limb anomalies, tall stature, CDH is rare	GPC3	Xp26.2	XL	+	Nk
Denys-Drash syndrome	194080	genital abnormalities, nephropathy, Wilms tumor, CDH is rare	WT1	11p13	AD	+	Nk
Frasier syndrome	136680	genital abnormalities, progressive nephrotic syndrome, gonadoblastoma, CDH is rare	WT1	11p13	AD	+	Nk
Meacham syndrome	608978	complex cardiovascular malformations, lung defects including severe pulmonary hypoplasia, genital abnormalities, CDH is rare	WT1	11p13	AD	+	Nk
WAGR syndrome	194072	Wilms tumor, aniridia, genitourinary anomalies, mental retardation, CDH is rare	WT1	11p13	AD	+	Nk
Apert syndrome	101200	craniosyntosis, mid-face hypoplasia, ocular hypertelorism, fusion of cervical vertebrae	FGFR2	10q26.13	AD	+	1 : 160.000

Syndrome	OMIM	Clinic	Gene	Locus	Inheritance	Molecular testing	Prevalence
Beckwith-Wiedemann syndrome	130650	abdominal wall defects, earlobe creases or pits behind the upper ear, macroglossia and visceromegaly, renal anomalies, hypoglycaemia, predisposition Wilms tumor and hepatoblastoma	CDKN1C, H19,LIT1 NSD1	11p15.5 5q35.2-q35.3	AD	+	1 : 13.700
CHARGE syndrome	214800	coloboma, cardiac defects, atresia choanae, retarded growth and development, genital hypoplasia, ear anomalies/deafness	CHD7 SEMA3E	8q12.1 7q21.11	AD	+	1 : 12.000
C syndrome (Trigonocephaly syndrome)	211750	metopic craniosynostosis, orofacial anomalies, genital anomalies, cardiovascular defects, short limbs	CD96	3q13.1-q13.2	AR	-	1 : 12.000
Coffin-Siris syndrome	135900	hypoplastic to absent fifth finger and toe nails, mental retardation	Nk	7q32-q34	AR	-	< 1 : 1.000.000
cutis laxa autosomal recessive type I	219100	loose redundant folds of the skin, pulmonary emphysema, aortic dilatation, pulmonary stenosis, cor pulmonale, diverticula, hernias	EFEMP2	11q13.1	AR	+	1-9 : 1.000.000
Czeizel-Losonci syndrome	183802	limb anomalies, urinary tract obstruction, neural tube defects	Nk	Nk	AD	-	Nk
Ehlers Danlos syndrome type 1	130000	loose-jointedness and fragile, bruisable skin that heals with peculiar 'cigarette-paper' scars	COL5A1 COL5A2 COL1A1	9q34.3 2q32.2 17q21.33	AD	+	1 : 5.000
Gershoni-Baruch syndrome	609545	omphalocele, cardiovascular malformations, absent radial ray, vertebral anomalies, neural tube defect	Nk	Nk	AR	-	Nk
Goltz syndrome (focal dermal hypoplasia)	305600	skin atrophy, multiple papillomas; digital, oral and ocular anomalies, osteopathia striata, male fetuses die already in utero	PORCN	Xp11.23	XL	+	Nk
Hemifacial microsomia	164210	facial asymmetry and ear anomalies, cardiac, vertebral, and central nervous system defects	Nk	14q32	AD	-	1 :3.000 - 5.000
Kabuki syndrome	147920	mental retardation, postnatal dwarfism, fingerpads, trapezoid philtrum, eversion of lower eyelids, large prominent ears	MLL2	12q12-q14	AD	+	1 : 32.000

Syndrome	OMIM	Clinic	Gene	Locus	Inheritance	Molecular testing	Prevalence
Marfan syndrome	154700	tall statue, disproportionately long extremities, subluxation of the lens, myopia, dilatation of the descending aorta	FBN1	15q21.1	AD	+	1 : 5.000–10.000
Mathieu syndrome	-	facial dysmorphology, cleft palate, short statue, short neck, vertebral abnormalities, tracheal abomalies	Nk	Nk	AD	-	Nk
MIDAS syndrome	309801	microphthalmia, dermal aplasia, sclerocornea	HCCS	Xp22.2	XL	+	< 1 : 1.000.000
Multiple pterygium syndrome Escobar variant	265000	webbing (pterygia) of the neck, elbows, and/or knees and joint contractures (arthrogryposis), skeletal defects and genital anomalies	CHRNG	2q37.1	AR	+	Nk
Myotubular myopathy 1	310400	generalized muscle weakness, congential eventration of the diaphragm	MTM1	Xq28	XL	+	1 :50.000
Opitz GBBB syndrome type 1	300000	hypertelorism, hypospadias, cleft lip/palate, laryngotracheoesophageal abnormalities, imperforate anus, developmental delay, cardiac defects	MID1	Xp22.2	XL	+	1-9 : 100.000
PAGOD syndrome	202660	agonadism, pulmonary hypoplasia, hypoplasia of pulmonary arteries, omphalocele/ diaphragmatic defects, dextrocardia	Nk	Nk	Nk	-	Nk
Pentalogy of Cantrell	313850	midline complex: thoraco abdominal syndrome, parasternal CDH	Nk	Nk	sporadic	-	5.5 : 1.000.000
Perlman syndrome	267000	nephroblastoma, fetal ascites, hamartoma, macrosomia, Wilms tumor	Nk	Nk	AR	-	Nk
Poland syndrome	173800	unilateral absence or hypoplasia of the pectoralis muscle, and a variable degree of ipsilateral hand and digit anomalies	Nk	Nk	Nk	-	1 – 3 : 100.000
Swyer syndrome 46,XY sex reversal 1	400044	partial or complete gonadal dysgenesis	SRY	Yp11.31	Nk	+	Nk
Thoracoabdominal syndrome	313850	adominal wall defect such as absent or hypoplastic abdominis rectus muscle, diaphragm defects, hypoplastic lung	Nk	Xq25-q26.1	XL	-	1-9 : 1.000.000

AD: autosomal dominant, AR: autosomal recessive, XL: X-linked, R: Research only, NK: unknown

Table 2. CDH and associated genetic syndromes.

7. Pre- and postnatal diagnostic workup

7.1 Diagnostic investigations

If the diagnosis of congenital CDH is made prenatally, a number of diagnostic steps should be offered to the patient. These steps may be helpful in classifying CDH as isolated or complex, the latter based on chromosmal imbalance or of syndromic origin. Important information can also be obtained from looking at the lung size, volume and dopplers. This information may be helpful in assessing survival and to make plans for the location and setting of the delivery.

7.2 Evaluation strategies: Suggested workup for CDH patients

- prenatal high resolution ultrasound for anomaly scanning of additional defects and fetal echocardiography by a fetal medicine specialist:
  - 1st trimester screening: nuchal translucency may be increased on ultrasound (Sebire et al., 1997).
  - 2nd trimester anomaly scanning: herniated viscera, position of the liver in the fetal thorax, absence of the normal position of the stomach bubble below the diaphragm, mediastinal shift (Stege et al., 2003; Tonks et al., 2004).
  - polyhydramnios due to compression of esophagus (Witters et al., 2001).
  - calculation of the lung-to-heart ratio (Fig. 1) as prognostic marker (Heling et al., 2005; Laudy et al., 2003; Lipshutz et al., 1997).
  - color flow Doppler for demonstrating abnormal position of umbilical and portal vein, identify right-sided hernias.
- MRI scan calculation of lung volumes using fast spin-echo MRI provides prognosis for degree of pulmonary hypoplasia and subsequent fetal outcome (Hubbard et al., 1997; Matsuoka et al., 2003).
- chest x-ray (neonatal): bowel gas is visible above the diaphragm, mediastinal shift.
- assessment by a trained clinical geneticist (clinical examination, family history): three-generation family history, other relatives with multiple congenital anomalies, infants who died in the perinatal period, consider examination of relatives, see medical reports.
- Chromosome analysis (karyotyping; ideally at minimum 550 bands):
  - prenatally: chorionic villus sampling or amniocentesis
  - postnatally: lymphocyte stimulated blood culture (non-lymphocyte-derived tissue for isochromosome 12p), when considering the diagnosis of isochromosome 12p, peripheral blood chromosome are often normal, the isochromosome 12 may be present in chromosome analyses performed on non-lymphocyte lineages such as skin fibroblasts, amniocytes, chorionic villi cells, can eventually be detected by aCGH on DNA extracted from peripheral blood.
- fluorescence in situ hybridisation (FISH), multiple color FISH.
- screening by MLPA (multiplex ligation-dependent probe amplification) for (sub) telomeric rearrangements.
- screening by high-resolution array-CGH (array-based comparative genomic hypridization): used to detect structural differences in the genome or copy number variations (CNVs), in the form of microdeletions or microduplications in prenatally diagnosed cases of CDH and postnatally patients with growth retardation, facial

dysmorphology and /or major and minor anomalies in conjuction with CDH (Kantarci et al., 2006; Le Caignec et al., 2005), targeted arrays are being developed, arrays targeting known CDH hotspots such as 15q26 are available.

- SNP based copy number analyses.
- specific mutation analysis when patients fitting the phenotype of one of the syndromes: molecular gene testing for non-syndromic causes of CDH are not available as single gene mutations are rarely found, research testing for a FOG2 mutation is available.
- banking of fetal / neonatal metaphase pellets, DNA, cell lines and parental DNA registration in an (inter)national database, storage of fetal blood for biochemical analysis.
- physical pediatric examination of the newborn: scaphoid abdomen, diminished breath sounds ipsilateral to the side of the hernia, displacement of the heart sounds contralateral to the hernia.
- autopsy, alternatively minimal invasive autopsy or post-mortem MRI, photographs, skeletal x-rays, skin biopsy for cell line development, storage of diaphragm- and lung tissues for future functional analysis.

8. Management at birth

- planned delivery >37 weeks gestation.
- primary intubation.
- correction of hypercapnae and pre-ductal hypoxemia, assuring end-organ perfusion.
- infants do not need to be rushed to surgery and benefit from stabilization of respiratory and cardiovascular status prior to diaphragmatic repair.
- minimal sedation and pressure support modes of ventilation, eventually high-frequency oscillatory ventilation (HFOV)
- critical cardiopulmonary deterioration: consider extra-corporeal membrane oxygenation (ECMO), unclear whether it improves survival of CDH
- ex-utero intrapartum treatment (EXIT)
- others (controversial): nitric oxide (NO) or phosphodiesterase inhibitors for treatment of pulmonary hypertension, delay of surgical repair, surfactant, perflubron, fetal surgery, tracheal occlusion by fetal endoscopic balloon placement (isolated CDH without chromosomal aberrations and a small LH ratio of <0.8).

9. Conclusion

Congenital diaphragmatic hernia is a common birth defect with an estimated incidence of 1:3000 in live births (Langham et al., 1996). Despite advances in therapy, morbidity and mortality remains high especially when associated anomalies are found. Although the etiology of most cases of CDH remains unknown, there is increasingly evidence that genetic factors play an important role in the development of CDH. We presented candidate genes and genetic loci which are known to be associated with CDH. Future research will provide more information about the genetic factors causing the development of CDH. This understanding will eventually help us to establish preventive strategies or improve therapeutic interventions for patients with CDH.

10. References

Abe, T.; Kinouchi, K.; Fukumitsu, K.; Sasaoka, N.; Taniguchi, A. & Kitamura, S. (2001). [Perioperative management of twins with prenatally diagnosed congenital diaphragmatic hernia]. *Masui*, Vol.50, No.4, (Apr), pp. 394-8

Ackerman, K.G.; Herron, B.J.; Vargas, S.O.; Huang, H.; Tevosian, S.G.; Kochilas, L.; Rao, C.; Pober, B.R.; Babiuk, R.P.; Epstein, J.A.; Greer, J.J. & Beier, D.R. (2005). Fog2 is required for normal diaphragm and lung development in mice and humans. *PLoS Genet*, Vol.1, No.1, (Jul), pp. 58-65

Ackerman, K.G.; Wang, J.; Luo, L.; Fujiwara, Y.; Orkin, S.H. & Beier, D.R. (2007). Gata4 is necessary for normal pulmonary lobar development. *Am J Respir Cell Mol Biol*, Vol.36, No.4, (Apr), pp. 391-7

Addor, M.C.; Stefanutti, D.; Farron, F.; Meinecke, P.; Lacombe, D.; Sarlangue, J.; Prescia, G. & Schorderet, D.F. (1995). "C" trigonocephaly syndrome with diaphragmnatic hernia. *Genet Couns*, Vol.6, No.2, pp. 113-20

Albanese, C.T.; Lopoo, J.; Goldstein, R.B.; Filly, R.A.; Feldstein, V.A.; Calen, P.W.; Jennings, R.W.; Farrell, J.A. & Harrison, M.R. (1998). Fetal liver position and perinatal outcome for congenital diaphragmatic hernia. *Prenat Diagn*, Vol.18, No.11, (Nov), pp. 1138-42

Antonius, T.; van Bon, B.; Eggink, A.; van der Burgt, I.; Noordam, K. & van Heijst, A. (2008). Denys-Drash syndrome and congenital diaphragmatic hernia: another case with the 1097G > A(Arg366His) mutation. *Am J Med Genet A*, Vol.146A, No.4, (Feb 15), pp. 496-9

Austin-Ward, E.D. & Taucher, S.C. (1999). Familial congenital diaphragmatic hernia: is an imprinting mechanism involved? *J Med Genet*, Vol.36, No.7, (Jul), pp. 578-9

Ayme, S.; Julian, C.; Gambarelli, D.; Mariotti, B.; Luciani, A.; Sudan, N.; Maurin, N.; Philip, N.; Serville, F.; Carles, D. & et al. (1989). Fryns syndrome: report on 8 new cases. *Clin Genet*, Vol.35, No.3, (Mar), pp. 191-201

Baglaj, M.; Spicer, R. & Ashworth, M. (1999). Unilateral agenesis of the diaphragm: a separate entity or an extremely large defect? *Pediatr Surg Int*, Vol.15, No.3-4, pp. 206-9

Beighton, P.; De Paepe, A.; Steinmann, B.; Tsipouras, P. & Wenstrup, R.J. (1998). Ehlers-Danlos syndromes: revised nosology, Villefranche, 1997. Ehlers-Danlos National Foundation (USA) and Ehlers-Danlos Support Group (UK). *Am J Med Genet*, Vol.77, No.1, (Apr 28), pp. 31-7

Benacerraf, B.R.; Miller, W.A. & Frigoletto, F.D., Jr. (1988). Sonographic detection of fetuses with trisomies 13 and 18: accuracy and limitations. *Am J Obstet Gynecol*, Vol.158, No.2, (Feb), pp. 404-9

Berkovitz, G.D.; Fechner, P.Y.; Zacur, H.W.; Rock, J.A.; Snyder, H.M., 3rd; Migeon, C.J. & Perlman, E.J. (1991). Clinical and pathologic spectrum of 46,XY gonadal dysgenesis: its relevance to the understanding of sex differentiation. *Medicine (Baltimore)*, Vol.70, No.6, (Nov), pp. 375-83

Beurskens, L.W.; Tibboel, D. & Steegers-Theunissen, R.P. (2009). Role of nutrition, lifestyle factors, and genes in the pathogenesis of congenital diaphragmatic hernia: human and animal studies. *Nutr Rev*, Vol.67, No.12, (Dec), pp. 719-30

Beurskens, L.W.; Tibboel, D.; Lindemans, J.; Duvekot, J.J.; Cohen-Overbeek, T.E.; Veenma, D.C.; de Klein, A.; Greer, J.J. & Steegers-Theunissen, R.P. (2010). Retinol status of newborn infants is associated with congenital diaphragmatic hernia. *Pediatrics*, Vol.126, No.4, (Oct), pp. 712-20

Biggio, J.R., Jr.; Descartes, M.D.; Carroll, A.J. & Holt, R.L. (2004). Congenital diaphragmatic hernia: is 15q26.1-26.2 a candidate locus? *Am J Med Genet A*, Vol.126A, No.2, (Apr 15), pp. 183-5

Bittmann, S.; Ulus, H. & Springer, A. (2004). Combined pentalogy of Cantrell with tetralogy of Fallot, gallbladder agenesis, and polysplenia: a case report. *J Pediatr Surg*, Vol.39, No.1, (Jan), pp. 107-9

Bleyl, S.B.; Moshrefi, A.; Shaw, G.M.; Saijoh, Y.; Schoenwolf, G.C.; Pennacchio, L.A. & Slavotinek, A.M. (2007). Candidate genes for congenital diaphragmatic hernia from animal models: sequencing of FOG2 and PDGFRalpha reveals rare variants in diaphragmatic hernia patients. *Eur J Hum Genet*, Vol.15, No.9, (Sep), pp. 950-8

Bohn, D. (2002). Congenital diaphragmatic hernia. *Am J Respir Crit Care Med*, Vol.166, No.7, (Oct 1), pp. 911-5

Carmi, R.; Barbash, A. & Mares, A.J. (1990). The thoracoabdominal syndrome (TAS): a new X-linked dominant disorder. *Am J Med Genet*, Vol.36, No.1, (May), pp. 109-14

Carter, M.T.; St Pierre, S.A.; Zackai, E.H.; Emanuel, B.S. & Boycott, K.M. (2009). Phenotypic delineation of Emanuel syndrome (supernumerary derivative 22 syndrome): Clinical features of 63 individuals. *Am J Med Genet A*, Vol.149A, No.8, (Aug), pp. 1712-21

Casaccia, G.; Mobili, L.; Braguglia, A.; Santoro, F. & Bagolan, P. (2006). Distal 4p microdeletion in a case of Wolf-Hirschhorn syndrome with congenital diaphragmatic hernia. *Birth Defects Res A Clin Mol Teratol*, Vol.76, No.3, (Mar), pp. 210-3

Casaccia, G.; Digilio, M.C.; Seymandi, P.L. & Bagolan, P. (2008). Congenital diaphragmatic hernia in CHARGE syndrome. *Pediatr Surg Int*, Vol.24, No.3, (Mar), pp. 375-8

Chao, A.S.; Cheng, P.J.; Hsueh, C. & Soong, Y.K. (1997). The detection of right-sided congenital diaphragmatic hernia in monozygotic twins on prenatal ultrasonography. *J Obstet Gynaecol Res*, Vol.23, No.2, (Apr), pp. 153-5

Chassaing, N.; Lacombe, D.; Carles, D.; Calvas, P.; Saura, R. & Bieth, E. (2003). Donnai-Barrow syndrome: four additional patients. *Am J Med Genet A*, Vol.121A, No.3, (Sep 1), pp. 258-62

Chitayat, D.; Sroka, H.; Keating, S.; Colby, R.S.; Ryan, G.; Toi, A.; Blaser, S.; Viero, S.; Devisme, L.; Boute-Benejean, O.; Manouvrier-Hanu, S.; Mortier, G.; Loeys, B.; Rauch, A. & Bitoun, P. (2007). The PDAC syndrome (pulmonary hypoplasia/agenesis, diaphragmatic hernia/eventration, anophthalmia/microphthalmia, and cardiac defect) (Spear syndrome, Matthew-Wood syndrome): report of eight cases including a living child and further evidence for autosomal recessive inheritance. *Am J Med Genet A*, Vol.143A, No.12, (Jun 15), pp. 1268-81

Cho, H.Y.; Lee, B.S.; Kang, C.H.; Kim, W.H.; Ha, I.S.; Cheong, H.I. & Choi, Y. (2006). Hydrothorax in a patient with Denys-Drash syndrome associated with a diaphragmatic defect. *Pediatr Nephrol*, Vol.21, No.12, (Dec), pp. 1909-12

Clark, R.D. & Fenner-Gonzales, M. (1989). Apparent Fryns syndrome in a boy with a tandem duplication of 1q24-31.2. *Am J Med Genet*, Vol.34, No.3, (Nov), pp. 422-6

Clugston, R.D.; Klattig, J.; Englert, C.; Clagett-Dame, M.; Martinovic, J.; Benachi, A. & Greer, J.J. (2006). Teratogen-induced, dietary and genetic models of congenital diaphragmatic hernia share a common mechanism of pathogenesis. *Am J Pathol*, Vol.169, No.5, (Nov), pp. 1541-9

Clugston, R.D.; Zhang, W. & Greer, J.J. (2008). Gene expression in the developing diaphragm: significance for congenital diaphragmatic hernia. *Am J Physiol Lung Cell Mol Physiol*, Vol.294, No.4, (Apr), pp. L665-75

Coffin, G.S. & Siris, E. (1970). Mental retardation with absent fifth fingernail and terminal phalanx. *Am J Dis Child*, Vol.119, No.5, (May), pp. 433-9

Cohen, M.S.; Rychik, J.; Bush, D.M.; Tian, Z.Y.; Howell, L.J.; Adzick, N.S.; Flake, A.W.; Johnson, M.P.; Spray, T.L. & Crombleholme, T.M. (2002). Influence of congenital heart disease on survival in children with congenital diaphragmatic hernia. *J Pediatr*, Vol.141, No.1, (Jul), pp. 25-30

Colvin, J.; Bower, C.; Dickinson, J.E. & Sokol, J. (2005). Outcomes of congenital diaphragmatic hernia: a population-based study in Western Australia. *Pediatrics*, Vol.116, No.3, (Sep), pp. e356-63

Czeizel, A. & Kovacs, M. (1985). A family study of congenital diaphragmatic defects. *Am J Med Genet*, Vol.21, No.1, (May), pp. 105-17

Czeizel, A. & Losonci, A. (1987). Split hand, obstructive urinary anomalies and spina bifida or diaphragmatic defect syndrome with autosomal dominant inheritance. *Hum Genet*, Vol.77, No.2, (Oct), pp. 203-4

David, T.J. & Illingworth, C.A. (1976). Diaphragmatic hernia in the south-west of England. *J Med Genet*, Vol.13, No.4, (Aug), pp. 253-62

Day, R. & Fryer, A. (2003). Diaphragmatic hernia and preaxial polydactyly in spondylothoracic dysplasia. *Clin Dysmorphol*, Vol.12, No.4, (Oct), pp. 277-8

de Jong, G.; Rossouw, R.A. & Retief, A.E. (1989). Ring chromosome 15 in a patient with features of Fryns' syndrome. *J Med Genet*, Vol.26, No.7, (Jul), pp. 469-70

Dean, J.C.; Couzin, D.A.; Gray, E.S.; Lloyd, D.J. & Stephen, G.S. (1991). Apparent Fryns' syndrome and aneuploidy: evidence for a disturbance of the midline developmental field. *Clin Genet*, Vol.40, No.5, (Nov), pp. 349-52

Denamur, E.; Bocquet, N.; Baudouin, V.; Da Silva, F.; Veitia, R.; Peuchmaur, M.; Elion, J.; Gubler, M.C.; Fellous, M.; Niaudet, P. & Loirat, C. (2000). WT1 splice-site mutations are rarely associated with primary steroid-resistant focal and segmental glomerulosclerosis. *Kidney Int*, Vol.57, No.5, (May), pp. 1868-72

Devriendt, K.; Deloof, E.; Moerman, P.; Legius, E.; Vanhole, C.; de Zegher, F.; Proesmans, W. & Devlieger, H. (1995). Diaphragmatic hernia in Denys-Drash syndrome. *Am J Med Genet*, Vol.57, No.1, (May 22), pp. 97-101

Dillon, E.; Renwick, M. & Wright, C. (2000). Congenital diaphragmatic herniation: antenatal detection and outcome. *Br J Radiol*, Vol.73, No.868, (Apr), pp. 360-5

Donadio, A.; Garavelli, L.; Banchini, G. & Neri, G. (2000). Kabuki syndrome and diaphragmatic defects: a frequent association in non-Asian patients? *Am J Med Genet*, Vol.91, No.2, (Mar 13), pp. 164-5

Donnai, D. & Barrow, M. (1993). Diaphragmatic hernia, exomphalos, absent corpus callosum, hypertelorism, myopia, and sensorineural deafness: a newly recognized autosomal recessive disorder? *Am J Med Genet*, Vol.47, No.5, (Oct 1), pp. 679-82

Doray, B.; Girard-Lemaire, F.; Gasser, B.; Baldauf, J.J.; De Geeter, B.; Spizzo, M.; Zeidan, C. & Flori, E. (2002). Pallister-Killian syndrome: difficulties of prenatal diagnosis. *Prenat Diagn*, Vol.22, No.6, (Jun), pp. 470-7

Dott, M.M.; Wong, L.Y. & Rasmussen, S.A. (2003). Population-based study of congenital diaphragmatic hernia: risk factors and survival in Metropolitan Atlanta, 1968-1999. *Birth Defects Res A Clin Mol Teratol*, Vol.67, No.4, (Apr), pp. 261-7

Eichelberger, M.R.; Kettrick, R.G.; Hoelzer, D.J.; Swedlow, D.B. & Schnaufer, L. (1980). Agenesis of the left diaphragm: surgical repair and physiologic consequences. *J Pediatr Surg*, Vol.15, No.4, (Aug), pp. 395-7

Enns, G.M.; Cox, V.A.; Goldstein, R.B.; Gibbs, D.L.; Harrison, M.R. & Golabi, M. (1998). Congenital diaphragmatic defects and associated syndromes, malformations, and chromosome anomalies: a retrospective study of 60 patients and literature review. *Am J Med Genet*, Vol.79, No.3, (Sep 23), pp. 215-25

Entezami, M.; Runkel, S.; Kunze, J.; Weitzel, H.K. & Becker, R. (1998). Prenatal diagnosis of a lethal multiple pterygium syndrome type II. Case report. *Fetal Diagn Ther*, Vol.13, No.1, (Jan-Feb), pp. 35-8

Franceschini, P.; Guala, A.; Licata, D.; Botta, G.; Flora, F.; Angeli, G.; Di Cara, G. & Franceschini, D. (2003). Gershoni-Baruch syndrome: report of a new family confirming autosomal recessive inheritance. *Am J Med Genet A*, Vol.122A, No.2, (Oct 1), pp. 174-9

Fryns, J.P.; Moerman, F.; Goddeeris, P.; Bossuyt, C. & Van den Berghe, H. (1979). A new lethal syndrome with cloudy corneae, diaphragmatic defects and distal limb deformities. *Hum Genet*, Vol.50, No.1, pp. 65-70

Gallot, D.; Laurichesse, H. & Lemery, D. (2003). Selective feticide in monochorionic twin pregnancies by ultrasound-guided umbilical cord occlusion. *Ultrasound Obstet Gynecol*, Vol.22, No.5, (Nov), pp. 484-8

Gencik, A.; Moser, H.; Gencikova, A. & Kehrer, B. (1982). Familial occurrence of congenital diaphragmatic defect in three families. *Helv Paediatr Acta*, Vol.37, No.3, (Jun), pp. 289-93

Genevieve, D.; Amiel, J.; Viot, G.; Le Merrer, M.; Sanlaville, D.; Urtizberea, A.; Gerard, M.; Munnich, A.; Cormier-Daire, V. & Lyonnet, S. (2004). Atypical findings in Kabuki syndrome: report of 8 patients in a series of 20 and review of the literature. *Am J Med Genet A*, Vol.129A, No.1, (Aug 15), pp. 64-8

Gershoni-Baruch, R.; Machoul, I.; Weiss, Y. & Blazer, S. (1990). Unknown syndrome: radial ray defects, omphalocele, diaphragmatic hernia, and hepatic cyst. *J Med Genet*, Vol.27, No.6, (Jun), pp. 403-4

Ghidini, A.; Sirtori, M.; Romero, R. & Hobbins, J.C. (1988). Prenatal diagnosis of pentalogy of Cantrell. *J Ultrasound Med*, Vol.7, No.10, (Oct), pp. 567-72

Gibbs, D.L.; Rice, H.E.; Farrell, J.A.; Adzick, N.S. & Harrison, M.R. (1997). Familial diaphragmatic agenesis: an autosomal-recessive syndrome with a poor prognosis. *J Pediatr Surg*, Vol.32, No.2, (Feb), pp. 366-8

Gillis, L.A.; McCallum, J.; Kaur, M.; DeScipio, C.; Yaeger, D.; Mariani, A.; Kline, A.D.; Li, H.H.; Devoto, M.; Jackson, L.G. & Krantz, I.D. (2004). NIPBL mutational analysis in 120 individuals with Cornelia de Lange syndrome and evaluation of genotype-phenotype correlations. *Am J Hum Genet*, Vol.75, No.4, (Oct), pp. 610-23

Greenberg, F.; Copeland, K. & Gresik, M.V. (1988). Expanding the spectrum of the Perlman syndrome. *Am J Med Genet*, Vol.29, No.4, (Apr), pp. 773-6

Greer, J.J.; Babiuk, R.P. & Thebaud, B. (2003). Etiology of congenital diaphragmatic hernia: the retinoid hypothesis. *Pediatr Res*, Vol.53, No.5, (May), pp. 726-30

Gripp, K.W.; Donnai, D.; Clericuzio, C.L.; McDonald-McGinn, D.M.; Guttenberg, M. & Zackai, E.H. (1997). Diaphragmatic hernia-exomphalos-hypertelorism syndrome: a new case and further evidence of autosomal recessive inheritance. *Am J Med Genet*, Vol.68, No.4, (Feb 11), pp. 441-4

Grogan, P.M.; Tanner, S.M.; Orstavik, K.H.; Knudsen, G.P.; Saperstein, D.S.; Vogel, H.; Barohn, R.J.; Herbelin, L.L.; McVey, A.L. & Katz, J.S. (2005). Myopathy with skeletal asymmetry and hemidiaphragm elevation is caused by myotubularin mutations. *Neurology*, Vol.64, No.9, (May 10), pp. 1638-40

Han, X.Y.; Wu, S.S.; Conway, D.H.; Pawel, B.R.; Punnett, H.H.; Martin, R.A. & de Chadarevian, J.P. (2000). Truncus arteriosus and other lethal internal anomalies in Goltz syndrome. *Am J Med Genet*, Vol.90, No.1, (Jan 3), pp. 45-8

Haspeslagh, M.; Fryns, J.P. & van den Berghe, H. (1984). The Coffin-Siris syndrome: report of a family and further delineation. *Clin Genet*, Vol.26, No.4, (Oct), pp. 374-8

Heling, K.S.; Wauer, R.R.; Hammer, H.; Bollmann, R. & Chaoui, R. (2005). Reliability of the lung-to-head ratio in predicting outcome and neonatal ventilation parameters in fetuses with congenital diaphragmatic hernia. *Ultrasound Obstet Gynecol*, Vol.25, No.2, (Feb), pp. 112-8

Holder, A.M.; Klaassens, M.; Tibboel, D.; de Klein, A.; Lee, B. & Scott, D.A. (2007). Genetic factors in congenital diaphragmatic hernia. *Am J Hum Genet*, Vol.80, No.5, (May), pp. 825-45

Hou, J.W. & Wang, T.R. (1999). Extreme Poland anomaly associated with congenital diaphragmatic hernia. *Eur J Pediatr*, Vol.158, No.5, (May), pp. 433-4

Hoyer, J.; Kraus, C.; Hammersen, G.; Geppert, J.P. & Rauch, A. (2009). Lethal cutis laxa with contractural arachnodactyly, overgrowth and soft tissue bleeding due to a novel homozygous fibulin-4 gene mutation. *Clin Genet*, Vol.76, No.3, (Sep), pp. 276-81

Hubbard, A.M.; Adzick, N.S.; Crombleholme, T.M. & Haselgrove, J.C. (1997). Left-sided congenital diaphragmatic hernia: value of prenatal MR imaging in preparation for fetal surgery. *Radiology*, Vol.203, No.3, (Jun), pp. 636-40

Hucthagowder, V.; Sausgruber, N.; Kim, K.H.; Angle, B.; Marmorstein, L.Y. & Urban, Z. (2006). Fibulin-4: a novel gene for an autosomal recessive cutis laxa syndrome. *Am J Hum Genet*, Vol.78, No.6, (Jun), pp. 1075-80

Jancelewicz, T.; Vu, L.T.; Keller, R.L.; Jelin, E.B.; Bratton, B.J.; Townsend, T.C. & Nobuhara, K.K. (2010). Outcomes of multigestational pregnancies affected by congenital diaphragmatic hernia. *J Pediatr Surg*, Vol.45, No.9, (Sep), pp. 1753-8

Kadir, R.A.; Hastings, R. & Economides, D.L. (1997). Prenatal diagnosis of supernumerary chromosome derivative (22) due to maternal balanced translocation in association with diaphragmatic hernia: a case report. *Prenat Diagn*, Vol.17, No.8, (Aug), pp. 761-4

Kantarci, S.; Casavant, D.; Prada, C.; Russell, M.; Byrne, J.; Haug, L.W.; Jennings, R.; Manning, S.; Blaise, F.; Boyd, T.K.; Fryns, J.P.; Holmes, L.B.; Donahoe, P.K.; Lee, C.; Kimonis, V. & Pober, B.R. (2006). Findings from aCGH in patients with congenital diaphragmatic hernia (CDH): a possible locus for Fryns syndrome. *Am J Med Genet A*, Vol.140, No.1, (Jan 1), pp. 17-23

Kantarci, S.; Al-Gazali, L.; Hill, R.S.; Donnai, D.; Black, G.C.; Bieth, E.; Chassaing, N.; Lacombe, D.; Devriendt, K.; Teebi, A.; Loscertales, M.; Robson, C.; Liu, T.; MacLaughlin, D.T.; Noonan, K.M.; Russell, M.K.; Walsh, C.A.; Donahoe, P.K. & Pober, B.R. (2007). Mutations in LRP2, which encodes the multiligand receptor megalin, cause Donnai-Barrow and facio-oculo-acoustico-renal syndromes. *Nat Genet*, Vol.39, No.8, (Aug), pp. 957-9

Kantarci, S.; Ackerman, K.G.; Russell, M.K.; Longoni, M.; Sougnez, C.; Noonan, K.M.; Hatchwell, E.; Zhang, X.; Pieretti Vanmarcke, R.; Anyane-Yeboa, K.; Dickman, P.; Wilson, J.; Donahoe, P.K. & Pober, B.R. (2010). Characterization of the chromosome 1q41q42.12 region, and the candidate gene DISP1, in patients with CDH. *Am J Med Genet A*, Vol.152A, No.10, (Oct), pp. 2493-504

Keijzer, R.; Liu, J.; Deimling, J.; Tibboel, D. & Post, M. (2000). Dual-hit hypothesis explains pulmonary hypoplasia in the nitrofen model of congenital diaphragmatic hernia. *Am J Pathol*, Vol.156, No.4, (Apr), pp. 1299-306

Kennerknecht, I.; Sorgo, W.; Oberhoffer, R.; Teller, W.M.; Mattfeldt, T.; Negri, G. & Vogel, W. (1993). Familial occurrence of agonadism and multiple internal malformations in phenotypically normal girls with 46,XY and 46,XX karyotypes, respectively: a new autosomal recessive syndrome. *Am J Med Genet*, Vol.47, No.8, (Dec 1), pp. 1166-70

Kent, A.; Simpson, E.; Ellwood, D. & Silink, M. (2004). 46,XY sex-reversal (Swyer syndrome) and congenital diaphragmatic hernia. *Am J Med Genet A*, Vol.131, No.1, (Nov 15), pp. 103-5

Killeen, O.G.; Kelehan, P. & Reardon, W. (2002). Double vagina with sex reversal, congenital diaphragmatic hernia, pulmonary and cardiac malformations--another case of Meacham syndrome. *Clin Dysmorphol*, Vol.11, No.1, (Jan), pp. 25-8

Klaassens, M.; van Dooren, M.; Eussen, H.J.; Douben, H.; den Dekker, A.T.; Lee, C.; Donahoe, P.K.; Galjaard, R.J.; Goemaere, N.; de Krijger, R.R.; Wouters, C.; Wauters, J.; Oostra, B.A.; Tibboel, D. & de Klein, A. (2005). Congenital diaphragmatic hernia and chromosome 15q26: determination of a candidate region by use of fluorescent in situ hybridization and array-based comparative genomic hybridization. *Am J Hum Genet*, Vol.76, No.5, (May), pp. 877-82

Klaassens, M.; Galjaard, R.J.; Scott, D.A.; Bruggenwirth, H.T.; van Opstal, D.; Fox, M.V.; Higgins, R.R.; Cohen-Overbeek, T.E.; Schoonderwaldt, E.M.; Lee, B.; Tibboel, D. & de Klein, A. (2007). Prenatal detection and outcome of congenital diaphragmatic hernia (CDH) associated with deletion of chromosome 15q26: two patients and review of the literature. *Am J Med Genet A*, Vol.143A, No.18, (Sep 15), pp. 2204-12

Klaassens, M.; de Klein, A. & Tibboel, D. (2009). The etiology of congenital diaphragmatic hernia: still largely unknown? *Eur J Med Genet*, Vol.52, No.5, (Sep-Oct), pp. 281-6

Kondo, S.; Schutte, B.C.; Richardson, R.J.; Bjork, B.C.; Knight, A.S.; Watanabe, Y.; Howard, E.; de Lima, R.L.; Daack-Hirsch, S.; Sander, A.; McDonald-McGinn, D.M.; Zackai, E.H.; Lammer, E.J.; Aylsworth, A.S.; Ardinger, H.H.; Lidral, A.C.; Pober, B.R.; Moreno, L.; Arcos-Burgos, M.; Valencia, C.; Houdayer, C.; Bahuau, M.; Moretti-Ferreira, D.; Richieri-Costa, A.; Dixon, M.J. & Murray, J.C. (2002). Mutations in IRF6 cause Van der Woude and popliteal pterygium syndromes. *Nat Genet*, Vol.32, No.2, (Oct), pp. 285-9

Krassikoff, N. & Sekhon, G.S. (1990). Terminal deletion of 6q and Fryns syndrome: a microdeletion/syndrome pair? *Am J Med Genet*, Vol.36, No.3, (Jul), pp. 363-4

Lally, K.P.; Lally, P.A.; Lasky, R.E.; Tibboel, D.; Jaksic, T.; Wilson, J.M.; Frenckner, B.; Van Meurs, K.P.; Bohn, D.J.; Davis, C.F. & Hirschl, R.B. (2007). Defect size determines survival in infants with congenital diaphragmatic hernia. *Pediatrics*, Vol.120, No.3, (Sep), pp. e651-7

Langham, M.R., Jr.; Kays, D.W.; Ledbetter, D.J.; Frentzen, B.; Sanford, L.L. & Richards, D.S. (1996). Congenital diaphragmatic hernia. Epidemiology and outcome. *Clin Perinatol*, Vol.23, No.4, (Dec), pp. 671-88

Laporte, J.; Hu, L.J.; Kretz, C.; Mandel, J.L.; Kioschis, P.; Coy, J.F.; Klauck, S.M.; Poustka, A. & Dahl, N. (1996). A gene mutated in X-linked myotubular myopathy defines a new putative tyrosine phosphatase family conserved in yeast. *Nat Genet*, Vol.13, No.2, (Jun), pp. 175-82

Laudy, J.A.; Van Gucht, M.; Van Dooren, M.F.; Wladimiroff, J.W. & Tibboel, D. (2003). Congenital diaphragmatic hernia: an evaluation of the prognostic value of the lung-to-head ratio and other prenatal parameters. *Prenat Diagn*, Vol.23, No.8, (Aug), pp. 634-9

Le Caignec, C.; Boceno, M.; Saugier-Veber, P.; Jacquemont, S.; Joubert, M.; David, A.; Frebourg, T. & Rival, J.M. (2005). Detection of genomic imbalances by array based comparative genomic hybridisation in fetuses with multiple malformations. *J Med Genet*, Vol.42, No.2, (Feb), pp. 121-8

Li, M.; Shuman, C.; Fei, Y.L.; Cutiongco, E.; Bender, H.A.; Stevens, C.; Wilkins-Haug, L.; Day-Salvatore, D.; Yong, S.L.; Geraghty, M.T.; Squire, J. & Weksberg, R. (2001). GPC3 mutation analysis in a spectrum of patients with overgrowth expands the phenotype of Simpson-Golabi-Behmel syndrome. *Am J Med Genet*, Vol.102, No.2, (Aug 1), pp. 161-8

Lin, A.E.; Pober, B.R.; Mullen, M.P. & Slavotinek, A.M. (2005). Cardiovascular malformations in Fryns syndrome: is there a pathogenic role for neural crest cells? *Am J Med Genet A*, Vol.139, No.3, (Dec 15), pp. 186-93

Lin, A.E.; Pober, B.R. & Adatia, I. (2007). Congenital diaphragmatic hernia and associated cardiovascular malformations: type, frequency, and impact on management. *Am J Med Genet C Semin Med Genet*, Vol.145C, No.2, (May 15), pp. 201-16

Lipshutz, G.S.; Albanese, C.T.; Feldstein, V.A.; Jennings, R.W.; Housley, H.T.; Beech, R.; Farrell, J.A. & Harrison, M.R. (1997). Prospective analysis of lung-to-head ratio predicts survival for patients with prenatally diagnosed congenital diaphragmatic hernia. *J Pediatr Surg*, Vol.32, No.11, (Nov), pp. 1634-6

Lucas Talan, M.; Garcia, L.; Cortiella, P.; Lopez Gil, V.; Perapoch, J. & Miranda, L. (1998). [Delivery of twins with diaphragmatic hernia]. *Rev Esp Anestesiol Reanim*, Vol.45, No.3, (Mar), pp. 114-5

Lurie, I.W. (2003). Where to look for the genes related to diaphragmatic hernia? *Genet Couns*, Vol.14, No.1, pp. 75-93

Macayran, J.F.; Doroshow, R.W.; Phillips, J.; Sinow, R.M.; Furst, B.A.; Smith, L.M. & Lin, H.J. (2002). PAGOD syndrome: eighth case and comparison to animal models of congenital vitamin A deficiency. *Am J Med Genet*, Vol.108, No.3, (Mar 15), pp. 229-34

Machado, A.P.; Ramalho, C.; Portugal, R.; Brandao, O.; Carvalho, B.; Carvalho, F.; Matias, A. & Montenegro, N. Concordance for bilateral congenital diaphragmatic hernia in a monozygotic dichorionic twin pair - first clinical report. *Fetal Diagn Ther*, Vol.27, No.2, pp. 106-9

Manouvrier-Hanu, S.; Devisme, L.; Vaast, P.; Boute-Benejean, O. & Farriaux, J.P. (1996). Fryns syndrome and erupted teeth in a 24-weeks-old fetus. *Genet Couns*, Vol.7, No.2, pp. 131-4

Manouvrier, S.; Espinasse, M.; Vaast, P.; Boute, O.; Farre, I.; Dupont, F.; Puech, F.; Gosselin, B. & Farriaux, J.P. (1996). Brachmann-de Lange syndrome: pre- and postnatal findings. *Am J Med Genet*, Vol.62, No.3, (Mar 29), pp. 268-73

Martinez-Frias, M.L.; Bermejo, E.; Felix, V.; Jimenez, N.; Gomez-Ullate, J.; Lopez, J.A.; Aparicio, P.; Ayala, A.; Gairi, J.M.; Galan, E.; Suarez, M.E.; Penas, A.; de Tapia, J.M.; Nieto, C. & de la Serna, E. (1998). [Brachmann-de-Lange syndrome in our population: clinical and epidemiological characteristics]. *An Esp Pediatr*, Vol.48, No.3, (Mar), pp. 293-8

Masturzo, B.; Kalache, K.D.; Cockell, A.; Pierro, A. & Rodeck, C.H. (2001). Prenatal diagnosis of an ectopic intrathoracic kidney in right-sided congenital diaphragmatic hernia using color Doppler ultrasonography. *Ultrasound Obstet Gynecol*, Vol.18, No.2, (Aug), pp. 173-4

Mathieu, M.; De Broca, A.; Bony, H. & Piussan, C. (1993). A familial syndrome with micrognathia, cleft palate, short neck and stature, vertebral anomalies and mental retardation. *Genet Couns*, Vol.4, No.4, pp. 299-303

Matsuoka, S.; Takeuchi, K.; Yamanaka, Y.; Kaji, Y.; Sugimura, K. & Maruo, T. (2003). Comparison of magnetic resonance imaging and ultrasonography in the prenatal diagnosis of congenital thoracic abnormalities. *Fetal Diagn Ther*, Vol.18, No.6, (Nov-Dec), pp. 447-53

McGillivray, B.C. & Lowry, R.B. (1977). Poland syndrome in British Columbia: incidence and reproductive experience of affected persons. *Am J Med Genet*, Vol.1, No.1, pp. 65-74

Meacham, L.R.; Winn, K.J.; Culler, F.L. & Parks, J.S. (1991). Double vagina, cardiac, pulmonary, and other genital malformations with 46,XY karyotype. *Am J Med Genet*, Vol.41, No.4, (Dec 15), pp. 478-81

Mishalany, H. & Gordo, J. (1986). Congenital diaphragmatic hernia in monozygotic twins. *J Pediatr Surg*, Vol.21, No.4, (Apr), pp. 372-4

Moerman, P.; Fryns, J.P.; Devlieger, H.; Van Assche, A. & Lauweryns, J. (1987). Congenital eventration of the diaphragm: an unusual cause of intractable neonatal respiratory distress with variable etiology. *Am J Med Genet*, Vol.27, No.1, (May), pp. 213-8

Moore, A.W.; Schedl, A.; McInnes, L.; Doyle, M.; Hecksher-Sorensen, J. & Hastie, N.D. (1998). YAC transgenic analysis reveals Wilms' tumour 1 gene activity in the proliferating coelomic epithelium, developing diaphragm and limb. *Mech Dev*, Vol.79, No.1-2, (Dec), pp. 169-84

Morgan, N.V.; Brueton, L.A.; Cox, P.; Greally, M.T.; Tolmie, J.; Pasha, S.; Aligianis, I.A.; van Bokhoven, H.; Marton, T.; Al-Gazali, L.; Morton, J.E.; Oley, C.; Johnson, C.A.; Trembath, R.C.; Brunner, H.G. & Maher, E.R. (2006). Mutations in the embryonal subunit of the acetylcholine receptor (CHRNG) cause lethal and Escobar variants of multiple pterygium syndrome. *Am J Hum Genet*, Vol.79, No.2, (Aug), pp. 390-5

Mowery-Rushton, P.A.; Stadler, M.P.; Kochmar, S.J.; McPherson, E.; Surti, U. & Hogge, W.A. (1997). The use of interphase FISH for prenatal diagnosis of Pallister-Killian syndrome. *Prenat Diagn*, Vol.17, No.3, (Mar), pp. 255-65

Neri, G.; Gurrieri, F.; Zanni, G. & Lin, A. (1998). Clinical and molecular aspects of the Simpson-Golabi-Behmel syndrome. *Am J Med Genet*, Vol.79, No.4, (Oct 2), pp. 279-83

Neville, H.L.; Jaksic, T.; Wilson, J.M.; Lally, P.A.; Hardin, W.D., Jr.; Hirschl, R.B.; Langham, M.R., Jr. & Lally, K.P. (2002). Fryns syndrome in children with congenital diaphragmatic hernia. *J Pediatr Surg*, Vol.37, No.12, (Dec), pp. 1685-7

Niikawa, N.; Matsuura, N.; Fukushima, Y.; Ohsawa, T. & Kajii, T. (1981). Kabuki make-up syndrome: a syndrome of mental retardation, unusual facies, large and protruding ears, and postnatal growth deficiency. *J Pediatr*, Vol.99, No.4, (Oct), pp. 565-9

Panda, B.; Rosenberg, V.; Cornfeld, D. & Stiller, R. (2009). Prenatal diagnosis of ectopic intrathoracic kidney in a fetus with a left diaphragmatic hernia. *J Clin Ultrasound*, Vol.37, No.1, (Jan), pp. 47-9

Parmar, R.C.; Tullu, M.S.; Bavdekar, S.B. & Borwankar, S.S. (2001). Morgagni hernia with Down syndrome: a rare association -- case report and review of literature. *J Postgrad Med*, Vol.47, No.3, (Jul-Sep), pp. 188-90

Pasutto, F.; Sticht, H.; Hammersen, G.; Gillessen-Kaesbach, G.; Fitzpatrick, D.R.; Nurnberg, G.; Brasch, F.; Schirmer-Zimmermann, H.; Tolmie, J.L.; Chitayat, D.; Houge, G.; Fernandez-Martinez, L.; Keating, S.; Mortier, G.; Hennekam, R.C.; von der Wense, A.; Slavotinek, A.; Meinecke, P.; Bitoun, P.; Becker, C.; Nurnberg, P.; Reis, A. & Rauch, A.

(2007). Mutations in STRA6 cause a broad spectrum of malformations including anophthalmia, congenital heart defects, diaphragmatic hernia, alveolar capillary dysplasia, lung hypoplasia, and mental retardation. *Am J Hum Genet*, Vol.80, No.3, (Mar), pp. 550-60

Perlman, M. (1986). Perlman syndrome: familial renal dysplasia with Wilms tumor, fetal gigantism, and multiple congenital anomalies. *Am J Med Genet*, Vol.25, No.4, (Dec), pp. 793-5

Pilia, G.; Hughes-Benzie, R.M.; MacKenzie, A.; Baybayan, P.; Chen, E.Y.; Huber, R.; Neri, G.; Cao, A.; Forabosco, A. & Schlessinger, D. (1996). Mutations in GPC3, a glypican gene, cause the Simpson-Golabi-Behmel overgrowth syndrome. *Nat Genet*, Vol.12, No.3, (Mar), pp. 241-7

Pober, B.R.; Russell, M.K. & Ackerman, K.G. (1993). Congenital Diaphragmatic Hernia Overview. pp.

Pober, B.R.; Lin, A.; Russell, M.; Ackerman, K.G.; Chakravorty, S.; Strauss, B.; Westgate, M.N.; Wilson, J.; Donahoe, P.K. & Holmes, L.B. (2005). Infants with Bochdalek diaphragmatic hernia: sibling precurrence and monozygotic twin discordance in a hospital-based malformation surveillance program. *Am J Med Genet A*, Vol.138A, No.2, (Oct 1), pp. 81-8

Pober, B.R. (2008). Genetic aspects of human congenital diaphragmatic hernia. *Clin Genet*, Vol.74, No.1, (Jul), pp. 1-15

Revencu, N.; Quenum, G.; Detaille, T.; Verellen, G.; De Paepe, A. & Verellen-Dumoulin, C. (2004). Congenital diaphragmatic eventration and bilateral uretero-hydronephrosis in a patient with neonatal Marfan syndrome caused by a mutation in exon 25 of the FBN1 gene and review of the literature. *Eur J Pediatr*, Vol.163, No.1, (Jan), pp. 33-7

Robert, E.; Kallen, B. & Harris, J. (1997). The epidemiology of diaphragmatic hernia. *Eur J Epidemiol*, Vol.13, No.6, (Sep), pp. 665-73

Rodriguez, L.M.; Garcia-Garcia, I.; Correa-Rivas, M.S. & Garcia-Fragoso, L. (2004). Pulmonary hypoplasia in Jarcho-Levin syndrome. *P R Health Sci J*, Vol.23, No.1, (Mar), pp. 65-7

Rollnick, B.R. & Kaye, C.I. (1983). Hemifacial microsomia and variants: pedigree data. *Am J Med Genet*, Vol.15, No.2, (Jun), pp. 233-53

Saavedra, D.; Richieri-Costa, A.; Guion-Almeida, M.L. & Cohen, M.M., Jr. (1996). Craniofrontonasal syndrome: study of 41 patients. *Am J Med Genet*, Vol.61, No.2, (Jan 11), pp. 147-51

Sakazume, S.; Okamoto, N.; Yamamoto, T.; Kurosawa, K.; Numabe, H.; Ohashi, Y.; Kako, Y.; Nagai, T. & Ohashi, H. (2007). GPC3 mutations in seven patients with Simpson-Golabi-Behmel syndrome. *Am J Med Genet A*, Vol.143A, No.15, (Aug 1), pp. 1703-7

Scott, D.A.; Cooper, M.L.; Stankiewicz, P.; Patel, A.; Potocki, L. & Cheung, S.W. (2005). Congenital diaphragmatic hernia in WAGR syndrome. *Am J Med Genet A*, Vol.134, No.4, (May 1), pp. 430-3

Sebire, N.J.; Snijders, R.J.; Davenport, M.; Greenough, A. & Nicolaides, K.H. (1997). Fetal nuchal translucency thickness at 10-14 weeks' gestation and congenital diaphragmatic hernia. *Obstet Gynecol*, Vol.90, No.6, (Dec), pp. 943-6

Sergi, C.; Schulze, B.R.; Hager, H.D.; Beedgen, B.; Zilow, E.; Linderkamp, O.; Otto, H.F. & Tariverdian, G. (1998). Wolf-Hirschhorn syndrome: case report and review of the chromosomal aberrations associated with diaphragmatic defects. *Pathologica*, Vol.90, No.3, (Jun), pp. 285-93

Shaffer, L.G.; Theisen, A.; Bejjani, B.A.; Ballif, B.C.; Aylsworth, A.S.; Lim, C.; McDonald, M.; Ellison, J.W.; Kostiner, D.; Saitta, S. & Shaikh, T. (2007). The discovery of microdeletion syndromes in the post-genomic era: review of the methodology and characterization of a new 1q41q42 microdeletion syndrome. *Genet Med,* Vol.9, No.9, (Sep), pp. 607-16

Shehata, S.M.; El-Banna, I.A.; Gaber, A.A. & El-Samongy, A.M. (2000). Spondylothoracic dysplasia with diaphragmatic defect: a case report with literature review. *Eur J Pediatr Surg,* Vol.10, No.5, (Oct), pp. 337-9

Skari, H.; Bjornland, K.; Haugen, G.; Egeland, T. & Emblem, R. (2000). Congenital diaphragmatic hernia: a meta-analysis of mortality factors. *J Pediatr Surg,* Vol.35, No.8, (Aug), pp. 1187-97

Slavotinek, A.M. (2004). Fryns syndrome: a review of the phenotype and diagnostic guidelines. *Am J Med Genet A,* Vol.124A, No.4, (Feb 1), pp. 427-33

Slavotinek, A.M. (2007). Single gene disorders associated with congenital diaphragmatic hernia. *Am J Med Genet C Semin Med Genet,* Vol.145C, No.2, (May 15), pp. 172-83

Snijders, R.J.M. & Nicolaides, K.H. (1996). *Fetal abnormalities* The Parthenon Publishing Group, 1-85070-610-7, London, UK

Song, A. & McLeary, M.S. (2000). MR imaging of pentalogy of Cantrell variant with an intact diaphragm and pericardium. *Pediatr Radiol,* Vol.30, No.9, (Sep), pp. 638-9

Stege, G.; Fenton, A. & Jaffray, B. (2003). Nihilism in the 1990s: the true mortality of congenital diaphragmatic hernia. *Pediatrics,* Vol.112, No.3 Pt 1, (Sep), pp. 532-5

Steiner, R.D.; St, J.D.P.; Hopkin, R.J.; Kozielski, R. & Bove, K.E. (2002). Combination of diaphragmatic eventration and microphthalmia/anophthalmia is probably nonrandom. *Am J Med Genet,* Vol.108, No.1, (Feb 15), pp. 45-50

Struthers, J.L.; Cuthbert, C.D. & Khalifa, M.M. (1999). Parental origin of the isochromosome 12p in Pallister-Killian syndrome: molecular analysis of one patient and review of the reported cases. *Am J Med Genet,* Vol.84, No.2, (May 21), pp. 111-5

Suri, M.; Kelehan, P.; O'Neill, D.; Vadeyar, S.; Grant, J.; Ahmed, S.F.; Tolmie, J.; McCann, E.; Lam, W.; Smith, S.; Fitzpatrick, D.; Hastie, N.D. & Reardon, W. (2007). WT1 mutations in Meacham syndrome suggest a coelomic mesothelial origin of the cardiac and diaphragmatic malformations. *Am J Med Genet A,* Vol.143A, No.19, (Oct 1), pp. 2312-20

Tongsong, T.; Sirichotiyakul, S.; Wanapirak, C. & Chanprapaph, P. (2002). Sonographic features of trisomy 18 at midpregnancy. *J Obstet Gynaecol Res,* Vol.28, No.5, (Oct), pp. 245-50

Tonks, A.; Wyldes, M.; Somerset, D.A.; Dent, K.; Abhyankar, A.; Bagchi, I.; Lander, A.; Roberts, E. & Kilby, M.D. (2004). Congenital malformations of the diaphragm: findings of the West Midlands Congenital Anomaly Register 1995 to 2000. *Prenat Diagn,* Vol.24, No.8, (Aug), pp. 596-604

Torfs, C.P.; Curry, C.J.; Bateson, T.F. & Honore, L.H. (1992). A population-based study of congenital diaphragmatic hernia. *Teratology,* Vol.46, No.6, (Dec), pp. 555-65

Toyama, W.M. (1972). Combined congenital defects of the anterior abdominal wall, sternum, diaphragm, pericardium, and heart: a case report and review of the syndrome. *Pediatrics,* Vol.50, No.5, (Nov), pp. 778-92

Turleau, C.; de Grouchy, J.; Chavin-Colin, F.; Martelli, H.; Voyer, M. & Charlas, R. (1984). Trisomy 11p15 and Beckwith-Wiedemann syndrome. A report of two cases. *Hum Genet,* Vol.67, No.2, pp. 219-21 van Dooren, M.F.; Brooks, A.S.; Tibboel, D. & Torfs, C.P. (2003). Association of congenital diaphragmatic hernia with limb-reduction defects. *Birth Defects Res A Clin Mol Teratol*, Vol.67, No.8, (Aug), pp. 578-84

Vasudevan, P.C.; Twigg, S.R.; Mulliken, J.B.; Cook, J.A.; Quarrell, O.W. & Wilkie, A.O. (2006). Expanding the phenotype of craniofrontonasal syndrome: two unrelated boys with EFNB1 mutations and congenital diaphragmatic hernia. *Eur J Hum Genet*, Vol.14, No.7, (Jul), pp. 884-7

Vissers, L.E.; van Ravenswaaij, C.M.; Admiraal, R.; Hurst, J.A.; de Vries, B.B.; Janssen, I.M.; van der Vliet, W.A.; Huys, E.H.; de Jong, P.J.; Hamel, B.C.; Schoenmakers, E.F.; Brunner, H.G.; Veltman, J.A. & van Kessel, A.G. (2004). Mutations in a new member of the chromodomain gene family cause CHARGE syndrome. *Nat Genet*, Vol.36, No.9, (Sep), pp. 955-7

Watanatittan, S. (1983). Congenital diaphragmatic hernia in identical twins. *J Pediatr Surg*, Vol.18, No.5, (Oct), pp. 628-9

Weksberg, R.; Shuman, C.; Caluseriu, O.; Smith, A.C.; Fei, Y.L.; Nishikawa, J.; Stockley, T.L.; Best, L.; Chitayat, D.; Olney, A.; Ives, E.; Schneider, A.; Bestor, T.H.; Li, M.; Sadowski, P. & Squire, J. (2002). Discordant KCNQ1OT1 imprinting in sets of monozygotic twins discordant for Beckwith-Wiedemann syndrome. *Hum Mol Genet*, Vol.11, No.11, (May 15), pp. 1317-25

Weksberg, R.; Shuman, C. & Beckwith, J.B. (2010). Beckwith-Wiedemann syndrome. *Eur J Hum Genet*, Vol.18, No.1, (Jan), pp. 8-14

Wieland, I.; Jakubiczka, S.; Muschke, P.; Cohen, M.; Thiele, H.; Gerlach, K.L.; Adams, R.H. & Wieacker, P. (2004). Mutations of the ephrin-B1 gene cause craniofrontonasal syndrome. *Am J Hum Genet*, Vol.74, No.6, (Jun), pp. 1209-15

Wimplinger, I.; Morleo, M.; Rosenberger, G.; Iaconis, D.; Orth, U.; Meinecke, P.; Lerer, I.; Ballabio, A.; Gal, A.; Franco, B. & Kutsche, K. (2006). Mutations of the mitochondrial holocytochrome c-type synthase in X-linked dominant microphthalmia with linear skin defects syndrome. *Am J Hum Genet*, Vol.79, No.5, (Nov), pp. 878-89

Witters, I.; Legius, E.; Moerman, P.; Deprest, J.; Van Schoubroeck, D.; Timmerman, D.; Van Assche, F.A. & Fryns, J.P. (2001). Associated malformations and chromosomal anomalies in 42 cases of prenatally diagnosed diaphragmatic hernia. *Am J Med Genet*, Vol.103, No.4, (Nov 1), pp. 278-82

Wolff, G. (1980). Familial congenital diaphragmatic defect: review and conclusions. *Hum Genet*, Vol.54, No.1, pp. 1-5

Zalis, E.G. & Roberts, D.C. (1967). Ehlers-Danlos syndrome with a hypoplastic kidney, bladder diverticulum, and diaphragmatic hernia. *Arch Dermatol*, Vol.96, No.5, (Nov), pp. 540-4

Zelante, L. & Ruscitto, M.M. (2003). Fusion of vertebrae, diaphragmatic hernia and unusual facies in a girl: a possible further case of Mathieu syndrome. *Clin Dysmorphol*, Vol.12, No.3, (Jul), pp. 207-8

6

Diagnosis of Congenital Diaphragmatic Hernia (CDH)

Kotis Alexandros, Tsikouris Panagiotis, Lisgos Philip, Dellaporta Irini, Georganas Marios, Ikonomidou Ioanna, Tsiopanou Eleni and Karatapanis Stylianos
General Hospital of Rhodes
Greece

1. Introduction

Congenital diaphragmatic hernia (CDH) is a congenital malformation (birth defect) of the diaphragm. The most common type of CDH is a Bochdalek hernia; other types include Morgagni's hernia, diaphragm eventration and central tendon defects of the diaphragm. Malformation of the diaphragm allows the abdominal organs to push into the chest thereby impeding proper lungformation. CDH is a life-threatening pathology in infants, and a major cause of death due to two complications: pulmonary hypoplasia and pulmonary hypertension. The frequency of CHD is approximately 1/3000 births. The survival rate for infants with hernias of the foramen of Bochdalek varies from institution to institution; but overall, it has remained at about 50% for nearly half a century, despite advances in neonatal intensive care, anesthesia, and surgery. CDH is believed to result from incomplete fusion of the pleuroperitoneal membrane, and passage of the abdominal contents into the chest. A chest x-ray can confirm the diagnosis if bowel gas is visible above the diaphragm accompanied by a mediastinal shift. CDH can also be found in older children (5-30% of CHD)(32) presenting with acute distress or GI symptoms, in most cases due to an episode of infection with involvement of the residual lung and airways (B streptococcus pneumonia) or posttraumatic involvement. This paper aims to evaluate the appearance of congenital diaphragmatic hernia (CDH) by diagnostic imaging methods.Anterior CHD through the foramen of Morgagni (90% right sided) is less common (1-5%) and is usually asymptomatic(31). Prenatal US and/or prenatal MRI already detects the hernia in utero in most cases(28). The intrathoracic space restriction results in ipsilateral lung hypoplasia. The associated pulmonary hypertension makes it very difficult to provide adequate oxygenation. Restoring the intrathoracic space and achieving pulmonary expansion are the main goals of surgery.

2. Diagnosis and testing

Congenital diaphragmatic hernia can be detected prenatally by an ultrasound examination performed during the second trimester in most affected infants.Clinical examination of the newborn with CDH often reveals a scaphoid abdomen (since the abdominal contents can be in the thorax), diminished breath sounds ipsilateral to the side of the hernia, and displacement of the heart sounds contralateral to the hernia. A chest x-ray can confirm the diagnosis if bowel gas is visible above the diaphragm accompanied by a mediastinal shift.

2.1

Diaphragmatic anomalies indirectly involve the gastrointestinal system by allowing herniation or displacement of abdominal contents into the thorax, thereby distorting normal anatomic relationships. The following diaphragmatic anomalies have been detected by antenatal sonography: posterolateral (Bochdalek) hernias, anterolateral (Morgagni) hernias, and diaphragmatic eventrations. Posterolateral diaphragmatic hernias are the most common and form as a result of incomplete fusion of the pneumoperitoneal membrane during embryogenesis. Occuring more frequently on the left than the right, they are typically associated with herniation of abdominal viscera such as stomach, spleen, and small bowel into the left hemithorax. Right-sided defects tend to involve the liver and gallbladder,so they may be more difficult to diagnose due to similarities in echogenicity of fetal lung and liver(27). Sonographic findings commonly identified in conjunction with posterolateral diaphragmatic hernias include cystic or solid intrathoracic masses corresponding to abdominal organs, mediastinal shift, smaller than expected abdominal circumference, and, failure to identify a fluid filled stomach in the left upper quadrant(25,26,27). Polyhydramnios is frequent and pleural effusions or ascites are occasionally seen. Paradoxical movement of the abdominal contents on the side of the hernia has been described during fetal respiratory efforts. Positive identification of intrathoracic bowel loops is possible when peristalsis is observed during real time evaluation. In the absence of this specific finding, documentation of a very low abdominal circumference or lack of gastric visualization is strongly suggestive of diaphragmatic hernia if seen in conjunction with unilateral thoracic mass lesions. Other fetal intrathoracic masses such as cystic adenomastoid malformation, pulmonary sequestration, and bronchogenic cyst should also be considered in the differential diagnosis. Although it is possible to overdiagnose diaphragmatic hernias on oblique scans that demonstrate thoracic and abdominal contents in the same plane, if care is taken to obtain a true cross section of the chest, this pitfall can be avoided. Even when peristalsis of intrathoracic bowel loops is observed, a definitive diagnosis of diaphragmatic hernia may not be possible because the sonographic findings associated with diaphragmatic eventration may be almost identical with those seen with hernias. In a recent series of diaphragmatic anomalies, detected antenatally, the only finding distinguishing a case of diaphragmatic eventration was a normal abdominal circumference. Although diaphragmatic hernias are usually accompanied by severe respiratory complications related to pulmonary hypoplasia, pulmonary function tends to be much better in infants with unilateral diaphragmatic eventration. Anteromedial (Morgagni) hernias form as a result of maldevelopment of the septum transversum in the retrosternal area. They are often associated with a defect in the pericardium, allowing abdominal contents to herniate into the pericardial sac. Antenatal sonography may reveal pericardial effusion and an anteriorly located intrathoracic mass in cases of anteromedial diaphragmatic hernia.(24)

Congenital abnormalities of the diaphragm range from total agenesis, an extreme life threatening condition with herniation of abdominal contents into the thorax, to that of a rare accessory hemidiaphragm that describes an almost vertical course through the chest, along the course of the major fissure, radiographically mimicking upper lobe disease or collapse, particularly on the left side(36). Eventrations (localized congenital weaknesses or absence of the musculature of the central portion of the diaphragm) usually manifest themselves as smooth convex mounds interrupting the gentle curvature of the diaphragm normally seen on chest radiographs. This most commonly presents in childhood on the right side, whereas that found in adults has a left-sided predominance. With eventration a curious tilting of the liver may be seen during the course of CT examination, where the anterior portion of that organ occupies a higher position than its posterior half. Both fluoroscopy and ultrasound may be used to evaluate the motion of the diaphragm in this condition. Very little or no inferior movement is seen on inspiration. The most common organ herniating through the hemidiaphragm is the stomach (36). The less common of the diaphragmatic hernias are those through the foramen of Morgagni anteromedially. These occur predominantly on the right and usually contain omentum; however, liver and colon are occasionally present within them. Herniation through an incompletely closed posterolateral pleuroperitoneal membrane (the foramen of Bochdalek) is usually on the left side. These are common in infants and may contain retroperitoneal fat, spleen, kidney or even large bowel. Congenital diaphragmatic hernia may be diagnosed prenatally using ultrasound, when the abdominal organs may be visualized within the fetal thorax, even displacing the mediastinum. In the newborn, respiratory distress, a scaphoid abdomen, and air-filled loops of bowel in one side of the chest usually suggest the diagnosis. In the case of bilateral anteromedial defects of the diaphragm, a characteristic picture of a three tiered snowman, with elevation of the heart and thymus by herniation of abdominal structures through a single midline opening, is usually seen(36).

The large diaphragmatic hernias that compromise lung growth are posterolateral in position and are caused by defective closure of the pleuroperitoneal canal. The remnant of this canal in the normally developed diaphragm is the foramen of Bochdalek. Typically, infants with congenital diaphragmatic hernias are severely distressed at birth, and because the abdomen contains fewer contents than normal, it appears scaphoid. Radiographically, the abdominal contents, which may include stomach, bowel, spleen and liver, can be identified within the thorax. Approximately 85% of congenital hernias are left sided(33).Rarely multicystic lesions such as cystic adenomatoid malformation may be considered in the differential diagnosis. In this situation fluoroscopy has been advocated in order to visualize intestinal peristalsis, but barium studies are not required. The ipsilateral lung is the more severely hypoplastic, but because of mediastinal shift, a lesser degree of contralateral hypoplasia is also present. The aerated ipsilateral lung may be visible preoperatively in the apex of the hemithorax, but the true degree of growth arrest can be appreciated only postoperatively when the tiny lung, tethered by the hilum, is outlined by a large pneumothorax. Contralateral hypoplasia is not as obvious, although more severe involvement may be indirectly indicated by the presence of pneumothorax caused by overdistention of underdeveloped alveoli. For this reason, the complication of contralateral pneumothorax signifies a poor prognosis(34).

The diaphragmatic hernia affects the lung primarily by interference with airway generation. Following unsuccessful operation, alveoli multiply at a normal rate and increase in size in an attempt to obtain normal lung volume. However airways are unable to multiply postnatally and there are also fewer pulmonary vessels. As it always increases in volume, the overdistended alveoli of the persistently hypoplastic lung result in a hyperlucent, emphysematous appearance, particularly of the lower lobe(35).

2.2

There is a high incidence of anomalies associated with each of the diaphragmatic lesions discussed here. These include chromosomal anomalies and gastrointestinal, genitourinary and cardiovascular defects. Identification of a diaphragmatic anomaly should prompt careful sonographic evaluation of the fetus for concomitant abnormalities as well as consideration of chromosomal analysis.In the absence of other lethal lesions, antenatal sonographic detection of diaphragmatic defects requires delivery to be performed at a tertiary care center appropriately equipped to manage the affected newborn, thus maximizing the infant's chance of survival.

2.3

Clinical examination is seldom revealing of a diagnosis, although a large rupture may mimic cardiac tamponade. The chest radiograph in the erect position may be the most diagnostic clue. Elevation of the hemidiaphragm, hemothorax, and bowel loops in the chest may lead one to perform upper and/or lower GI tract barium examinations, ultrasound, CT, angiography of the celiac axis, liver and lung scans, or even administration of contrast through a chest tube with a search for its appearance in the abdomen(36). CXR or ultrasound scan will confirm the diagnosis in a neonate who has not previously been diagnosed. Arterial blood gas measurements are required for pH, $PaCO_2$ and PaO_2. With persistent pulmonary hypertension with right-to-left ductal shunting, the PaO_2 may be higher from a pre-ductal (right-hand) sampling site. Blood samples must be monitored for electrolytes, calcium and glucose. Ultrasound of the heart and urinary system may be required to assess for other abnormalities.Cranial ultrasonography will highlight neural abnormalities such as hydrocephalus and neural tube defects. Chromosomal analysis may be indicated.(22).

2.4

Additionally air-fluid loops of bowel in a congenital diaphragmatic hernia can resemble the multiple cysts of cystic adenomatoid malformation. An important clue to the correct diagnosis of diaphragmatic hernia is the absence or paucity of gas-filled bowel loops within the abdomen. Congenital diaphragmatic hernias most often occur through the foramen of Bochdalek, which lies posteriorly and medially in each hemidiaphragm. Left-sided hernias are more common and more frequently involve bowel herniation. Solid abdominal viscera are more likely to herniate into the chest through right-sided hernias. Hernias through the foramen of Morgagni, which lies anteriorly, are less common and usually are less severe. Infants with large diaphragmatic hernias usually present with severe respiratory distress immediately after birth. Compression of the ipsilateral lung in utero causes it to be hypoplastic and often the contralateral lung is also small. The patients are profoundly hypoxic and a persistent fetal circulation caused by hypoxia -induced pulmonary hypertension usually further compromises the infant's condition. Even with early diagnosis and surgery, the mortality of this condition remains high. ECMO has improved the survival of some patients by circumventing the problem of pulmonary hypertension and the right-to left shunting of blood away from the lungs. Congenital diaphragmatic hernia may be minimally symptomatic at birth and can present later in life(20).

Poor outcomes have been connected with pneumothorax (reflecting lung hypoplasia) and a right-sided defect, whereas favorable features include the presence of aerated ipsilateral lung and aeration in the contralateral lung of more than 50%.

Congenital diaphragmatic hernia (CDH) is a major surgical emergency in newborns and the key to survival lies in prompt diagnosis and treatment.

From many imaging studies Aspelund et al concluded that prenatal LHR > 0.85 predicts survival for infants with isolated left-sided CDH without compromising discrimination of survivors from non-survivors. The diagnostic utility of LHR may be confounded by gestational age at measurement. Stringent LHR threshold may minimize false-negative attribution and improve utility of this measurement as predictor of survival. Kozakiewitz et al concluded that congenital diaphragmatic hernia (CDH) in most cases presents immediately or within hours after birth with signs of respiratory failure: dyspnea, tachypnea, and cyanosis. Kline-farh et al concluded that with further research with prenatal US and fetal MRI and the development of innovative medical and surgical therapies, the morbidity and mortality of children with congenital diaphragmatic hernias can be significantly reduced. Cruz-Martinez et al concluded that Intrapulmonary artery Doppler evaluation helps to refine the prediction of survival after FETO in fetuses with severe CDH and that the minimum number of scans required for an inexperienced trainee to become competent in examining the LHR is on average 70. Cannie M et al concluded that there is a significant relationship between Apparent Diffusion Coefficient (low) and Apparent Diffusion Coefficient (high) values and gestational age in normal fetal lungs. This relationship is most probably explained by developmental changes during the last three stages of lung development, which involve intense peripheral growth of airways and vessels as well as maturation. In CDH, measurement of ADC (low) might be useful as a predictor of postnatal outcome that is independent of lung volume.Gorincour G, et al concluded that normal fetal lung signal intensity curves can be obtained. Lungs at risk of hypoplasia presented significant alterations of signal ratios. The prognostic value of such results requires additional postnatal clinical follow-up. Kilian et al concluded that among fetuses with left-sided CDH, assessment of pulmonary hypoplasia based on MRI relative fetal lung volume and MRI relative lung-to-head ratio is excellent in prediction of neonatal survival and ECMO requirement. The prognostic accuracy is slightly better than that of sonographic relative lung-to-head ratio. Among fetuses with right-sided CDH, the prognostic value of all parameters is lower than those among fetuses with left-sided defects. Jani J, et al concluded that in the assessment of fetuses with CDH, MRI-based o/e Total Fetal Lung Volume is useful in the prediction of postnatal survival

Siegel MJ, et al in a study with seven patients with left-sided congenital diaphragmatic hernias at ages of 2-20 months are reported and five are described in detail. Radiographic findings were classic in one patient, but simulated inflammatory chest disease in two patients, gastric volvulus in three patients, and a pneumothorax in one patient. These misleading appearances if not recognized can lead to incorrect radiographic interpretation and in some cases inappropriate treatment. Reither M. concluded that the most common causes of respiratory distress in the newborn and the frequently rapidly changing pulmonary pattern in the follow up studies are presented. Various degrees of the hyaline membrane disease and bronchopulmonary dysplasia are demonstrated as well as the different changes of the pulmonary pattern in controlled and assisted ventilation, recurrent atelectasis, dystelectasis, emphysema, pneumothorax and pneumomediastinum. Chest film follow up series are demonstrated. The differential diagnosis includes pulmonary aspiration syndrome, the neonatal pneumonia and emergency cases in pediatric surgery. Hubbard AM et al demonstrated that in these fetuses, MR imaging proved important by clearly demonstrating herniation of fetal liver into the chest, thereby changing family counseling and prenatal care. Levin D. et al concluded that although oligohydramnios subjectively degrades image resolution, sonography still reveals important fetal anatomic landmarks. Major anomalies can be detected on sonography even when the pregnancy has less than the normal amount of amniotic fluid. Strouse PJ et al concluded that Congenital abnormalities of the umbilical venous system are rare. A case of fatal right congenital diaphragmatic hernia (CDH) in association with an anomalous umbilical vein bypassing the liver and directly entering the right atrium is presented. The ductus venosus was absent. Although much of the liver was within the right hemithorax, radiographs showed an apparently normal umbilical venous catheter (UVC) course, suggesting a normally positioned liver and mitigating against the diagnosis of CDH. Aberrant umbilical drainage, yielding a falsely normal appearing UVC course, may delay the diagnosis of CDH.Perez CG, demonstrated that Ultrasonographic examination of the fetal abdomen is an integral part in all routine fetal sonograms and can provide significant information about the status and prognosis of the fetus. Although many types of fetal anomalies can be identified (i.e., gastroschisis, omphalocele, or congenital diaphragmatic hernia), there are several sonographic findings that are not clearly anomalous, but may be associated with poor fetal outcome. Echogenic fetal bowel, small or absent fetal stomach and fetal intra-abdominal calcifications all fall into this category. This article reviews the recent literature as it relates to these topics, including suggestions regarding the need for further action, and the types of further actions that are available to help identify abnormal fetuses and prevent unnecessary and/or invasive testing of normal ones. Urban BA,concluded that Helical CT amniography is an efficient means for evaluation of congenital diaphragmatic hernia. Accurate diagnosis was made in all three patients. Hubbard AM, et al concluded that MR imaging is a valuable adjunct to US for prenatal diagnosis of fetal chest masses. The need for immediate postnatal diagnosis has been de-emphasized, but the demand for precision and efficiency in preoperative cross-sectional imaging, monitoring progress and complications of treatment, and assistance with nutritional support has increased (Schwartz DS, et al.). Five cases with congenital diaphragmatic hernia all demonstrated fetal breathing activity by thoracic wall movement (Fox HE et al). In four of the fetuses, perinasal fluid flow was seen by the Doppler technique. The fetus with no demonstrated perinasal flow during breathing movements died in the early neonatal period and had pulmonary hypoplasia. Observation of the fetal breathing-related nasal and oropharyngeal fluid flow in cases of antenatally diagnosed congenital diaphragmatic hernia provides a rationale to hypothesize that the absence of this phenomenon is a useful marker for prenatal prediction of pulmonary hypoplasia. Guibaud L et al concluded that Sonography is highly accurate for prenatal diagnosis od CDH. Sonography also assists the prognostication of postnatal outcome in isolated CDH by allowing quantification of the contralateral lung area on a four-chamber view.

Knox E,et al demonstrated that in CDH, LHR and the presence of liver in the fetal thorax may be a useful predictive indicator of perinatal survival. Future usage of developing techniques needs careful evaluation prior to usage to guide therapy. Mullassery D, et al demonstrated that Liver herniation is associated with poorer prognosis in fetal CDH. Grading liver herniation or using it as part of a panel of markers may enhance the value of liver herniation as a prognostic test in fetal CDH. Bagłaj M, et al concluded that Chest radiography following passage of a nasogastric tube and contrast studies of the gastrointestinal tract seem to be the most useful investigations for the diagnosis of left CDH. For patients with right CDH, owing to the high probability of liver herniation, a chest radiograph with liver scintigraphy or CT seems to be the best diagnostic option. Coleman BG, et al demonstrated that Fetal therapy is a rapidly evolving specialty, which is being practiced at several centers in this country. Sonography is an integral part of this specialty practice and has been used extensively in the diagnosis of some congenital anomalies that have debilitating or lethal consequences for the fetus. Technologic improvements in both sonography and magnetic resonance imaging have assisted tremendously in the many advances herein reported in the diagnosis and treatment of the above-described 4 congenital anomalies. Coakley FV. Et al showed that prenatal MRI has been shown to positively and incrementally influence management in a substantial proportion of patients being considered for fetal intervention. Despite these findings, precise indications for prenatal MRI in the setting of fetal surgery are not yet established, because both prenatal MRI and fetal surgery are relatively new techniques that remain in evolution. Fox HE, et al showed that all studies show that there is a clear association between most of these markers and pulmonary hypoplasia. However, these markers have not been studied together in a large number of cases, and comparisons between each of the markers is unknown

3. Imaging studies

Radiography

3.1

In the neonatal and infantile periods, the importance of obtaining a chest radiograph at the first sign of distress cannot be overstated. This image usually permits an accurate diagnosis, alternatively sometimes plain abdominal radiography is also needed for a precise diagnosis. Typically, no bowel gas is evident in the abdomen. A chest x-ray can confirm the diagnosis if bowel gas is visible above the diaphragm accompanied by a mediastinal shift. Congenital diaphragmatic hernia can be detected prenatally by an ultrasound examination performed during the second trimester in most affected infants

3.2

In patients presenting in the neonatal and infantile periods, the classic radiographic appearance of congenital diaphragmatic hernia is one in which the left hemithorax is filled with loops of bowel, the mediastinum is shifted to the right, and the abdomen is relatively devoid of gas. In some cases, a few loops of intestine can be seen in the abdomen, but more often only the stomach remains visible within the abdomen. Interestingly, the stomach may be in an abnormal location, often more central than one would expect. The abnormal positioning of the stomach may be helpful in differentiating congenital diaphragmatic hernia from those few cases of congenital cystic adenomatoid malformation (CCAM) in which the cysts are large enough to mimic the air-filled intestinal loops. In CCAM of the lungs, the stomach and bowel are normal in position and appearance.

3.3

If the chest radiograph is obtained before any air has entered the herniated bowel, diagnosing this condition with accuracy may be difficult. Similar difficulties arise when the liver alone is in the right hemithorax. In either case, the involved hemithorax is partially or totally opacified, and the mediastinal structures are shifted to the other side. In this circumstance, a large pleural fluid collection or mass may be present; however, in most such cases, air soon enters the intestine, and this finding establishes the diagnosis. In other cases, the condition may be diagnosed by noting abnormal intrathoracic positioning of a nasogastric tube.

3.4

Placement of an orogastric tube prior to the study helps decompress the stomach and helps determine whether the tube is positioned above or below the diaphragm.

3.5

Typical findings in a left-sided posterolateral congenital diaphragmatic hernia include air-filled or fluid-filled loops of the bowel in the left hemithorax and shift of the cardiac silhouette to the right. Examine the chest radiograph for evidence of pneumothorax. The incidence of associated cardiac anomalies is high (approximately 25%); therefore, cardiac ultrasonography is needed shortly after birth. Cardiac defects may be relatively minor (atrial septal defect) or life-threatening (transposition of great vessels, hypoplastic left heart, aortic coarctation). In addition, echocardiography is helpful in assessing myocardial function and determining whether the left ventricular mass is significantly decreased(18,19). Unusual findings on plain radiography include a contralateral pneumothorax, contralateral collapse/consolidation, fluid in the chest, and the absence of a contralateral aerated lung. If herniation occurs on the right, the intestine and liver or the liver alone may fill the right hemithorax. If the liver is in the chest, its normal silhouette is not generally seen in the abdomen.

4. Morgagni hernias

4.1

Classically, Morgagni hernias appear as unilateral, mediastinal, and basal masses containing a variety of abdominal organs, including air-filled loops of intestine. Occasionally, these hernias may be bilateral, and in rare cases, they may produce significant respiratory distress. Large anterior-central diaphragmatic hernias may produce elevation of the cardiac silhouette and bilateral bulges to either side of the lower mediastinum. Often, these herniations occur into the pericardial cavity. When this occurs, serious cardio respiratory compromise can result.

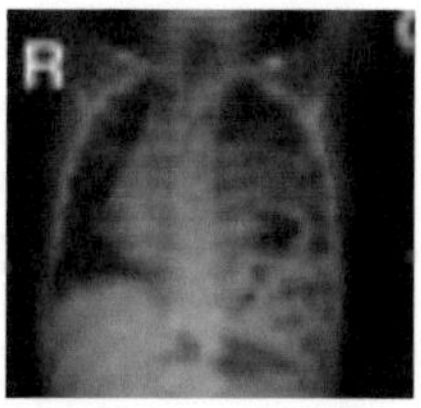

A 4 month old baby boy with congenital diaphragmatic hernia.

5. Computed tomography

5.1

In adults with congenital diaphragmatic hernia, previously undiagnosed Bochdalek hernias are most frequently identified when patients undergo computed tomography (CT) scanning for reasons that appear to be unrelated to the hernia. These Bochdalek hernias usually contain retroperitoneal fat or a kidney. Some authors believe that, with the routine use of thin-section CT scanning on modern imaging equipment, the prevalence and characteristics of late-presenting Bochdalek hernia can be more accurately estimated. However, small Bochdalek defects may occur in as many as 6% of older adults. Additionally was marked improvement over conventional CT amniography in embryos with helical CT amniography. Data are obtained immediately after localization with a low-dose topogram that eliminates the need for real-time sonographic guidance(21).

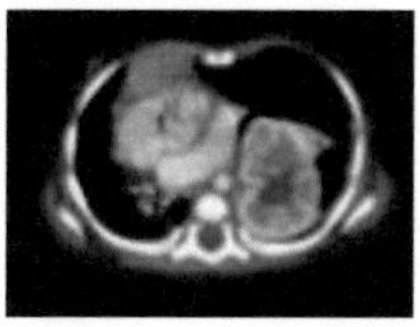

A 4 month old baby boy with congenital diaphragmatic hernia.

6. Magnetic resonance imaging

6.1

Regarding the prenatal magnetic resonance imaging (MRI) evaluation of congenital diaphragmatic hernia, advances in this modality provide high-quality images of the intrathoracic organs. MRIs can clearly depict diaphragmatic discontinuity, a fetal compressed lung, and connecting bowel segments between the abdomen and chest. MRI can accurately depict congenital diaphragmatic hernia and permits an easy diagnosis. MRI findings can be used to differentiate this condition from other chest masses, and MRI is superior to ultrasonography in demonstrating the position of the fetal liver above or below the diaphragm. Fetal MRI is increasingly being used to confirm the diagnosis of CDH, as well as to better define the internal anatomy [Hedrick et al 2004]. Calculation of lung volumes using fast spin-echo MRI appears to provide good prognosis about the degree of pulmonary hypoplasia and subsequent fetal outcome and seems likely to replace the LHR derived from ultrasound examination for this purpose [Gorincour et al 2005](17). Ultrafast fetal MRI – an imaging technique advanced at CHOP that checks the position of the abdominal organs, especially the liver, and measures protrusion into the chest. Ultrafast fetal MRI is used to better define the severity of CDH, exclude associated anomalies and estimate fetal lung volume as a prognostic indicator. We recommend fetal MRI two times during gestation. The first MRI is obtained during the initial evaluation in order to demonstrate the anatomic defect and determine whether or not the liver is herniated, which may be difficult to determine with ultrasound alone. Fetal MRI is useful in excluding other associated abnormalities in the chest, abdomen and brain. Magnetic Resonance Imaging (MRI) testing can assist in these efforts as well. Sometimes CDH does not appear through ultrasound images, and a diagnosis is made after the child has been born. There are a few centers where a Fetal Therapeutic or CDH team might both evaluate a baby prior to birth, and discuss treatment options with the parents of the child. Fetal MRI is increasingly being used to confirm the diagnosis of CDH, as well as to better define the internal anatomy [Hedrick et al 2004]. Calculation of lung volumes using fast spin-echo MRI appears to provide good prognosis about the degree of pulmonary hypoplasia and subsequent fetal outcome and seems likely to replace the LHR derived from ultrasound examination for this purpose [Gorincour et al 2005].

When CDH is found on routine prenatal ultrasound examination, both a high-resolution ultrasound examination and fetal MRI to determine the presence of additional structural anomalies are indicated. Chromosome analysis of fetal cells obtained by amniocentesis should be considered in all cases while CGH should strongly be considered when CDH is present in conjunction with additional anomalies.

All fetuses with CDH should be evaluated for the presence of syndromes and/or additional major malformations given that they so commonly coexist and significantly affect the prognosis. Involvement of a medical geneticist in the evaluation of these families can be helpful. The measurement of either the expected/observed LHR or the lung volume by fetal MRI have been useful to predict outcome; however, since the predictive value of these measurements varies from center to center, results must be interpreted with caution.

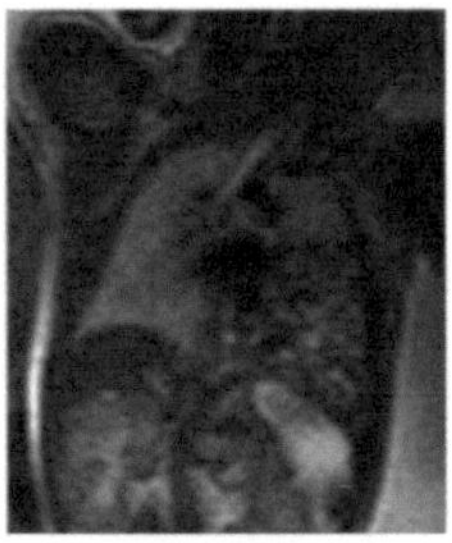

Fig. 1. 34-week fetus with left-sided congenital diaphragmatic hernia.

7. Ultrasonography

7.1

In prenatal life, ultrasonography has a high sensitivity in the detection of congenital diaphragmatic hernia. Bowel loops may appear to undergo peristalsis in the chest. The definite ultrasonographic diagnosis of fetal congenital diaphragmatic hernia lies on the visualization of abdominal organs in the chest; the ultrasonographic hallmark of this condition is a fluid-filled mass just behind the left atrium and ventricle in the lower thorax, as seen on a transverse view. In patients presenting in the prenatal period, ultrasonographic features indicative of congenital diaphragmatic hernia include polyhydramnios, an absent or intrathoracic stomach bubble, a mediastinal and cardiac shift away from the side of the herniation, a small fetal abdominal circumference, the absence of the stomach in the abdomen, and, rarely, fetal hydrops.In a right-sided hernia, the right lobe of the liver alone may be herniated, or associated hydrothorax and ascites may be observed. Pregnant women carrying a fetus with congenital diaphragmatic hernia are often referred for ultrasonography first because of suspected polyhydramnios. **Color flow Doppler** can be used to: Demonstrate abnormal positioning of the umbilical and portal veins, which are indicative of liver herniation; Identify right-sided hernias, which can be difficult to detect on ultrasound examination because of the similar echogenicity of lung and liver(16). As with other birth defects, most congenital diaphragramatic hernias (CDHs) are typically discovered by routine ultrasound at 16 to 18 weeks gestation. Families referred to The Children's Hospital of Philadelphia's Center for Fetal Diagnosis and Treatment undergo a comprehensive, one-day evaluation that includes: High-definition level II ultrasound – to assess the defect and to determine the fetus' lung-to-head circumference ratio (LHR), a measure that can help predict the severity of lung problems associated with CDHM any infants are now diagnosed in utero by Ultrasound imaging testing often identifies CDH before the child is born. Further ultrasound testing, once the fetus has been diagnosed with CDH, can help to determine the severity of the disorder and any additional problems that may be present.Chest x-Ray in CHD is frequently abnormal but not always diagnostic. A"bubbly"hemithorax with obliteration of the costophrenic sinus,deviation of the mediastinum to the controlateral side, abnormal position of the nasogastric tube,and an airless abdomen are the most common findings on chest and abdominal X-ray(28,29). Sometimes differential diagnosis with aerated congenital cystic adenomatoid malformation (CCAM) is equivocal. In these cases US can help in further diagnosis:the presence of mobile gastrointestinal structures and spleen,in severe cases parts of the liver confirms the hernia(28,29,30). Diaphragmatic eventration is usually the result of congenital paralysis,aplasia,or atrophy of the diaphragmatic muscle,and is seen on chest X-ray as an abnormally elevated diaphragm,partly or totally(31). Left-sided eventrations are more likely to be complete. The severity of presentation depends on the location and whether it involves a complete leaflet(31). Rarely,diaphragmatic eventration is bilateral and can lead to respiratory distress in infants,especially when associated with infection.

Ultrasound examination. The majority of infants with CDH are now diagnosed prenatally by ultrasound examination, which demonstrates herniated viscera with or without liver in the fetal thorax, absence of the normal position of the stomach bubble below the diaphragm, and mediastinal shift [Stege et al 2003, Tonks et al 2004]. Although not specific for CDH, polyhydramnios is often detected [Witters et al 2001].Calculation of the lung-to-head ratio (LHR) may be of prognostic value; however, centers have reported mixed results in the utility of this measure for predicting fetal outcome [Lipshutz et al 1997, Laudy et al 2003, Heling et al 2005]. Specifically, the "size" of the right lung is compared to the head circumference; a high ratio (>1.4) indicates good lung size and predicts a good outcome; a low ratio (variously cited as <1.0 or <0.6) indicates small lung size and predicts a poor outcome [Lipshutz et al 1997, Laudy et al 2003]. Some of the limitations of use of the LHR for predicting outcome:

- Inter-observer variability in determining the LHR is considerable.
- An indeterminate ratio between 1.0 and 1.4 is found in most fetuses.
- Prognostic accuracy is reduced for the following: right-sided CDH, additional birth defects, and/or diagnosis before 24 weeks gestation or after 26 weeks gestation.

Note: Gestational age is expressed as menstrual weeks calculated either from the first day of the last normal menstrual period or by ultrasound measurements.

Color flow Doppler can be used to:

- Demonstrate abnormal positioning of the umbilical and portal veins, which are indicative of liver herniation;
- Identify right-sided hernias, which can be difficult to detect on ultrasound examination because of the similar echogenicity of lung and liver.

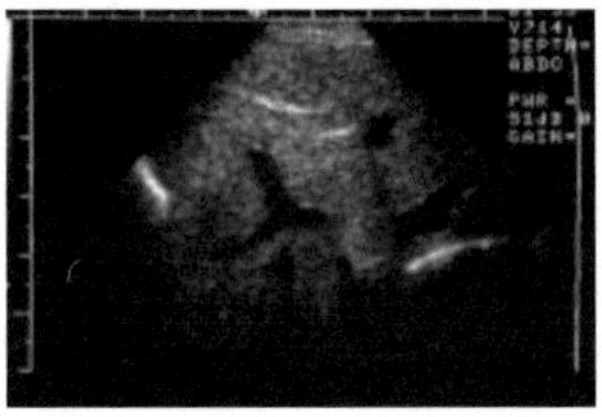

Ultrasonogram of a right-sided congenital diaphragmatic hernia shows the liver herniating through the defect.

8. References

[1] Saifuddin A, Arthur RJ. Congenital diaphragmatic hernia--a review of pre- and postoperative chest radiology. *Clin Radiol*. Feb 1993;47(2):104-10.

[2] Gale ME. Bochdalek hernia: prevalence and CT characteristics. *Radiology*. Aug 1985;156(2):449-52.

[3] Mullins ME, Stein J, Saini SS, Mueller PR. Prevalence of incidental Bochdalek's hernia in a large adult population. *AJR Am J Roentgenol*. Aug 2001;177(2):363-6.

[4] Reed JO, Lang EF. Diaphragmatic hernia in infancy. *Am J Roentgenol Radium TherNucl Med*. Sep 1959;82:437-49.

[5] Mitanchez D. [Antenatal treatment of congenital diaphragmatic hernia: An update.]. *Arch Pediatr*. Jun 27 2008;

[6] Pelizzo G, Lembo MA, Franchella A. Gastric volvulus associated with congenital diaphragmatic hernia, wandering spleen, and intrathoracic left kidney: CT findings. *Abdom Imaging*. May-Jun 2001;26(3):306-8.

[7] Swischuk LE. Imaging of the Newborn, Infant and Young Child. *4th ed*. Lippincott Williams & Wilkins;1997:68-72, 398-99, 412-23.

[8] Tibboel D, Gaag AV. Etiologic and genetic factors in congenital diaphragmatic hernia. *ClinPerinatol*. Dec 1996;23(4):689-99.

[9] Wilcox DT, Irish MS, Holm BA, Glick PL. Prenatal diagnosis of congenital diaphragmatic hernia with predictors of mortality. *ClinPerinatol*. Dec 1996;23(4):701-9.

[10] Cannie M, Jani J, De Keyzer F, Van Kerkhove F, Meersschaert J, Lewi L, et al. Magnetic resonance imaging of the fetal lung: a pictorial essay. *EurRadiol*. Jul 2008;18(7):1364-74.

[11] Shin SM, Mulligan SA, Baxley WA, HO KJ. Bochdalek Hernia of Diaphragm in the Adult: Diagnosis by Computed Tomography. Chest 1987;92:1098-1101

[12] Diaphragmatic Rupture Due to BluntTrauma: Sensitivity of Plain Chest Radiographs. AJR 1991;156:51-57

[13] Sergio G Golombek MD, FAAP Perinatology (2002) 22, 242-246 DOI: 10.1038/sj/jp/7210701The History of Congenital Diaphragmatic Hernia from 1850s to the Present.

[14] Keith A. On the origin and nature of hernia. Br J Surg 1924; 11: 455..

[15] Prenatal prediction of neonatal morbidity in survivors with congenital diaphragmatic hernia: a multicenter study. Ultrasound Obstet Gynecol. 2008 Oct 9. PMID: 18844275

[16] Masturzo B, Kalache KD, Cockell A, Pierro A, Rodeck CH. Prenatal diagnosis of an ectopic intrathoracic kidney in right-sided congenital diaphragmatic hernia using color Doppler ultrasonography. Ultrasound Obstet Gynecol. 2001;18:173–4. [PubMed: 11530002]

[17] Gorincour G, Bouvenot J, Mourot MG, Sonigo P, Chaumoitre K, Garel C, Guibaud L, Rypens F, Avni F, Cassart M, Maugey-Laulom B, Bourliere-Najean B, Brunelle F, Durand C, Eurin D. Prenatal prognosis of congenital diaphragmatic hernia using magnetic resonance imaging measurement of fetal lung volume. Ultrasound Obstet Gynecol. 2005;26:738–44. [PubMed: 16273597]

[18] Gross RE. Congenital hernia of the diaphragm.*Am J Dis Child*. 1946;71:579-592.

[19] Areechon W, Reid L. Hypoplasia of the lung associated with congenital diaphragmatic hernia. *Br Med J*. 1963;i:230-3.

[20] Brant WE: Pulmonarycavities. In Brant WE,Helms CA(eds): Fundamentals of Diagnostic Radiology 2nded. Baltimore, Lippincott Williams & Wilkins 2007 pp 1240-41

[21] Kelly DR,Grant EG, Zeman RK, Choyke PL, Bolan JC, Warsof SL. In utero diagnosis of congenital diaphragmatic hernia by CT amniography J Comput Assist Tomogr 1986;10:500-502

[22] Doyle NM, Lally KP; The CDH Study Group and advances in the clinical care of the patient with congenital diaphragmatic hernia. SeminPerinatol. 2004 Jun;28(3):174-84.

[23] *Thomas C. Weiss* - Published: 2009-01-28

[24] Comstock CH: The antenatal diagnosis of diaphragmatic anomalies, J Ultrasound Met 5-391,1986

[25] Barss VA, Benacerraf BR, Frigoletto FD: Antenatalsonographic diagnosis of fetal gastrointestinal malformations.Pediatrics76:445.1985

[26] Benacerraf BR, Greene MF: Congenital diaphragmatic hernia: US diagnosis prior to 22 weeks gestation.Radiology 158:809,1986

[27] Chinn DH, Filly RA, Callen PW, et al: Congenital diaphragmatic hernia diagnosed prenatally by ultrasound Radiology 148:119.1983

[28] Gibson AT, Steiner GM (1997) Imaging of the neonatal chest.ClinRadiol 52:172-186

[29] Alford BA, Mcllhenny J, Jones JE, Sutton CL, Silen M, Rodgers BM, McKinney CD(1993) Assymetric radiographic findings in the pediatric chest:approach to early diagnosis,Radiographics 13:77-93

[30] Rencken I, Patton WL, Brasch RC (1998) Airway obstruction in pediatric patients.RadiolClin North Am 36;175-187

[31] Singh S, Behnde MS, Kinnane GM, (2001) Delayed presentations of congenital diaphragmatic hernia. PediatrEmerg Care 17:269-271

[32] Schafermeyer R(1993) Pediatric trauma. Emerg Med Clin North Am 11:187-251

[33] Bonham Carter RE, Waterston DJ, Aberdeen E: Hernia and eventration of the diaphragm in childhood.Lancet 1:656,1962

[34] Fliegel CP, Kaufmann HJ; Problems caused my pneumothorax in congenital diaphragmatic hernia. Ann Radiol 15;159,1972

[35] Berdon WE, Baker DH, Amoury R: The role of pulmonary hyoplasia in the prognosis of newborn infants with diaphragmatic hernia and eventration AJR 103:413,1968

[36] Putman CH and Ravin C. Textbook of diagnostic Imaging 2nd EdsCh 41Chest Wall and hemidiaphragm 1994

[37] Lipshutz GS, Albanese CT, Feldstein VA, Jennings RW, Housley HT, Beech R, Farrell JA, Harrison MR. Prospective analysis of lung-to-head ratio predicts survival for patients with prenatally diagnosed congenital diaphragmatic hernia. J Pediatr Surg. 1997;32:1634–6. [PubMed: 9396544]

[38] Laudy JA, Van Gucht M, Van Dooren MF, Wladimiroff JW, Tibboel D. Congenital diaphragmatic hernia: an evaluation of the prognostic value of the lung-to-head ratio and other prenatal parameters. PrenatDiagn. 2003;23:634–9. [PubMed: 12913869]

[39] Stege G, Fenton A, Jaffray B. Nihilism in the 1990s: the true mortality of congenital diaphragmatic hernia. Pediatrics. 2003;112:532–5. [PubMed: 12949279]

[40] Tonks A, Wyldes M, Somerset DA, Dent K, Abhyankar A, Bagchi I, Lander A, Roberts E, Kilby MD. Congenital malformations of the diaphragm: findings of the West Midlands Congenital Anomaly Register 1995 to 2000. PrenatDiagn. 2004;24:596–604. [PubMed: 15305345]

[41] Witters I, Legius E, Moerman P, Deprest J, Van Schoubroeck D, Timmerman D, Van Assche FA, Fryns JP. Associated malformations and chromosomal anomalies in 42 cases of prenatally diagnosed diaphragmatic hernia.Am J Med Genet. 2001;103:278–82. [PubMed: 11746006]

[42] Heling KS, Wauer RR, Hammer H, Bollmann R, Chaoui R. Reliability of the lung-to-head ratio in predicting outcome and neonatal ventilation parameters in fetuses with congenital diaphragmatic hernia. Ultrasound Obstet Gynecol. 2005;25:112–8. [PubMed: 15660446]

[43] Hedrick HL, Crombleholme TM, Flake AW, Nance ML, von Allmen D, Howell LJ, Johnson MP, Wilson RD, Adzick NS. Right congenital diaphragmatic hernia: Prenatal assessment and outcome. J Pediatr Surg. 2004;39:319–23. [PubMed:15017545]

[44] Gorincour G, Bouvenot J, Mourot MG, Sonigo P, Chaumoitre K, Garel C, Guibaud L, Rypens F, Avni F, Cassart M, Maugey-Laulom B, Bourliere-Najean B, Brunelle F, Durand C, Eurin D. Prenatal prognosis of congenital diaphragmatic hernia using magnetic resonance imaging measurement of fetal lung volume. Ultrasound Obstet Gynecol. 2005;26:738–44. [PubMed]

Section 3

Management of Congenital Diaphragmatic Hernia

7

Congenital Diaphragmatic Hernia and Associated Anomalies

Milind Joshi, Sharad Khandelwal, Priti Zade and Ram Milan Prajapati
SAIMS, Indore
India

1. Introduction

Congenital diaphragmatic hernia (CDH) is associated with multiple reported associated anomalies. Knowledge of these anomalies and their management if required should be part of overall treatment. Many of these are fatal and have known association with chromosomal abnormalities and can result in still born babies. Another aspect of the knowledge of these anomalies is in predicting the recurrence in the subsequent pregnancies.

The key determinants of mortality are whether the CDH is isolated or complex, co existence of major anomalies, size of the diaphragm defect, degree of pulmonary hypoplasia, severity of pulmonary hypertension in the perinatal period, side of the hernial defect. The major morbidity associated with CDH are pulmonary, gastro intestinal, neurological, musculoskeletal, hearing loss (1).

It has been well established that disruption of the retinoic acid signaling pathway is associated with development of CDH [(1)]. There is evidence that retinoic acid and vitamin A play an important role in the development of diaphragm and other aspects of organogenesis. However, it is difficult to explain the role of vitamin A in cases of isolated CDH. One small study showed decreased levels of retinol in the newborns with CDH compared to controls (2).

The reported incidence of CDH is between 1 in 2000 to 5000 births (3). The incidence of still births is not well documented but about one third of these babies are still born. The deaths are due to associated fatal congenital anomalies. Bilateral CDH are associated with high incidence of associated anomalies than the unilateral one (4). Infants with isolated CDH are more likely to be premature and macrosomic and male.

About one third of the patients have major congenital malformation (5). Although CDH is thought to be a sporadic developmental anomaly familial cases have been reported and recurrence risk in a first degree relative has been estimated to be about 2%. Chromosomal anomalies have been reported to occur in 9 to 34% patients common being trisomies, deletion and translocation. The combination of CDH and associated abnormal karyotype has been associated with a poor outcome. The incidence of associated malformations in CDH patients is about 10-50%.

2. Chromosomal abnormalities

About 10% of all individuals with CDH have a chromosome abnormality. The most common abnormalities are trisomy 18 and isochromosome 12p (6).

2.1 Chromosome 12p (Pallister Killian syndrome)

The presence of supernumerary isochromosome, with double copy of short arm of chromosome 12 is confirmatory. Isochromosomal mosaicism is the cardinal finding in this syndrome. This is commonly found in the infants born to the mothers of advanced age. The spectrum of the clinical problems in this syndrome ranges from multiple malformations incompatible with life to milder phenotypes.

The documented abnormalities include CDH, relatively shortened limb, CNS anomalies and ventricular dilatation, craniofacial dysmorphism, presence of nuchal skin edema, hydrops or poly hydromnios (7).

The typical facial dysmorphism include brachycephaly, high broad forehead, ocular hypertelorism, low set ears, broad nasal bridge, anteverted nostrils, long filtrum. Patients have normal growth and most patients have at least moderate intellectual disability. The distinguishing features from Fryns syndrome are the non hereditary nature, rare occurrence of nail hypoplasia which is one of the hallmark for Fryns syndrome (8).

Patients with Fryns syndrome have CDH, cleft palate, distal phalangeal and or nail hypoplasia, cardiovascular and renal malformations.

2.2 Trisomy 21

Infants with trisomy 21 can have Bochdalek or Morgagni hernia. It can be seen in association with presence of right sided diaphragmatic hernia or diaphragmatic eventration. (9).

2.3 Wolf Hirschhorn syndrome

This is characterized by deletion of distal portion of short arm of chromosome 4. It is possible that gene responsible for development of the diaphragm is deleted because there is very common association of this syndrome with CDH (10). The various other reported genetic syndromes are trisomy 18 and trisomy 22 (11).

2.4 Single gene disorders

Some of the more common single gene disorders in which CDH occurs are Cornelia de Lange syndrome, Denys Drash syndrome, Donnai Barrow syndrome, Fryns syndrome, spondylocoastal dysostosis, Meachan syndrome (8,12,13,14).

3. Malformations seen in non syndromic CDH

At least 33% of the CDH patients have associated major congenital malformations, commonly cardiovascular and pulmonary, central nervous, musculoskeletal.

3.1 Cardiovascular malformations

About one fourth of the patients with CDH have cardiovascular malformations. The most common malformations are ventricular septal defects and atrial septal defects.

The less commonly documented are Fallot's Tetralogy, hypoplastic left heart syndrome and dextrocardia, transposition of great vessels, double outlet of right ventricle and aortic coarctation. Anatomic anomalies of the tracheobronchial tree have been found in 18% of the patients. Congenital tracheal stenosis, tracheal bronchus and trifurgated trachea are reported (15).

3.2 Central nervous system abnormalities

This is the most common associated abnormality in fetuses stillborn with CDH. The most commonly diagnosed are neural tube defects, hydrocephalus (16,17) and rarely corpus callosum agenesis. The presence of sensorineural hearing loss also forms the part of the associated anomalies.

3.3 Musculoskeletal abnormalities

The incidence is about 10% non syndromic CDH. The common occurrence limb reduction defects, polydactyly, syndactyly, hypoplastic thumb and Polland syndrome. This syndrome is associated with hypoplastic ribs on one side along with absence of ipsilateral pectoralis minor muscles (18,19,20,21,22).

3.4 Genitourinary abnormalities

Undescended or ectopic testis, thoracic ectopic kidney (23,24), ectopic kidney, horse shoe kidney are reported in the literature. Gonadal aplasia and hypoplasia, ambiguity have also been reported with CDH.

3.5 Gastro intestinal malformations

The common associations are malrotation, atresia, omphalocele and rarely situs ambiguous. Presence of abnormal gastroesophageal reflux and esophageal dysmotility is very common. Improper fixation of the ligaments of the stomach and subsequent volvulus of the stomach are also known in patients of CDH(25). Presence of Cantrell's Penta logy is one of the classical associations. This association is presence of anterior diaphragmatic hernia with, omphalocele, bifid sternum, ectopia cordis and congenital heart defects as ventricular septal defects and ventricular dilatation(25).

4. References

Brennan P, Croaker GD, Heath M: Congenital diaphragmatic hernia and interstitial deletion of chromosome 3. J Med Genet 2001;38:556-557.

Clugston RD, ZhangW, Alvarez S, de Lera AR et al. Understanding abnormal retinoid signaling as a causative mechanism in congenital diaphragmatic hernia. Am J Respir Cell Mol Biol 2010; 42: 272-285.

Cohen MS, Rychik J, Bush DM, Tian ZY et al. Influence of congenital heart disease on survival in children with congenital diaphragmatic hernia. J Pediatr 2002; 141:25- 30.

Dott MM, Wong LY, Rasmussen SA. Population based study of congenital diaphragmatic hernia : risk factors and survival in metripolital Atlanta, 1968-1999. Birth defects Res A Clin Mol Teratol. 2003; 67:267-269.

Day R, Fryer A. Diaphagmatic hernia and preaxial polydactyly in spondylothoracic dysplasia. Clin Dysmorphol. 2003;12: 277-278.

Friedman S, Chen C, Chapman J et al. Neurodevelopmental outcomes of congenital diaphragmatic hernia survivors in a multidisciplinary clinic at ages 1 and 3. J Pediatr Surg. 2008; 43; 1035-1046.

Joshi M, Parelkar S, Shah H et al. Acute gastric volvulus in children: 6 years experience at a single centre. Afr Jour Pediatr Surg. 2010; 22: 22-24.

Losty PD, Vanamo K, Rintala RJ et al. Congenital diaphragmatic hernia - does the side of the defect influence the incidence of associated malformations? J Pediatr Surg 1998; 33: 507-512.

Lurie IW. Where to look for genes related to diaphragmatic hernia? Genet Couns 2003; 14:75-78.

Kantarci S, Casavant D, PradaC et al. Findings from ACGH in patients with congenital diaphragmatic hernia: a possible locus for Fryns syndrome. Am J Med Genet A. 2006; 140:17-23.

Kantarci S, Al-Gazali L, Hill R et al. Mutataions in LRP2, which encodes the multiligand receptor megalin, cause Donnai Barrow and facio –oculo- acoustico- renal syndromes. Nat Genet. 2007; 39: 957-959.

Klaassens M, Scott D, van Dooren M et al. congenital diaphragmatic hernia associated with duplication of 11q 23 qter. Am J Med Genet A. 2006; 140: 1580-1586. 13. Masturzo B, Kalache KD, Cockell A. Prenatal diagnosis of ectopic intrathoracic kidney in right sided congenital diaphragmatic hernia using color Doppler ultrasonography. Ultrasound Obstet Gynecol. 2001; 18: 173-174.

Major D, Cadenas M, Fournier L et al. Retinol status of new born infants with congenital diaphragmatic hernia. Pediatr Surg Int. 1998; 13: 547-549.

Miagliazza L, Otten C, Xia H et al. cardiovascular malformations associated with congenital diaphragmatic hernia: experimental and human studies. J Pediatr Surg. 1999; 34: 1352-1357.

Miagliazza L, Xia H, Diez –Pardo JA et al. Skeletal malformations associated with congenital diaphragmatic hernia : experimental and human studies. J Pediatr Surg.1999; 34: 1624-1629.

Neville HL, Jaksic T, Wilson JM et al. Congenital diaphragmatic hernia study group: bilateral congenital diaphragmatic hernia. J Pediatr Surg. 2003; 38: 522- 524.

Nose K, Kamata S, Sawai T et al. Airway anomalies in patients with congenital diaphragmatic hernia. J Pediatr Surg. 2000; 35: 1562-1565.

Panda B, Rosenberg V, Cornfeld D. Prenatal diagnosis of ectopic intrathoracic kidney in a fetus with left sided diaphragmatic hernia. J Clin Ultrasound. 2009; 37: 47-49.

Sergi C, Schulze BR, Hager HD et al. Wolfe Hirsch Horn syndrome: case report and review of the chromosomal aberrations associated with congenital diaphragmatic defects. Pathologica. 1998; 90: 285-293.

Slavotinek AM. Fryns syndrome: a review of the phenotype and the diagnostic guidelines. Am J Med Genet A. 2004; 124A: 427-433.

Skari H, Bjornland K, Frencker B et al. Congenital diaphragmatic hernia: a meta analysis of mortality factors. J Pediatr Surg. 2000; 35: 1187-1197.

Van Dooren MF, Brooks AS, Tibbboel D et al. Association of congenital diaphragmatic hernia with limb reduction defects. Birth defects Res A Clin Mol Teratol. 2003; 67: 578- 584.

Witters I, Leguis E, Moerman P et al. Associated malformations and chromosomal anomalies in 42 cases of prenatally diagnosed diaphragmatic hernia. Am J Med Genet 2001 ; 103: 278- 280.

Yamataka T, Puri P. Pulmonary artery structural changes in pulmonary hypertension complicating congenital diaphragmatic hernia. J Pediatr Surg. 1997; 32: 387- 390.

8

Congenital Diaphragmatic Hernia and Congenital Heart Disease

Katey Armstrong[1,2,4], Orla Franklin[2] and Eleanor J. Molloy[1,3,4]
[1]*Paediatrics, National Maternity Hospital, Holles St., Dublin*
[2]*Paediatric Cardiology, Our Lady's Children's Hospital, Crumlin, Dublin*
[3]*Department of Paediatrics, Royal College of Surgeons of Ireland*
[4]*National Children's Research Centre, Dublin*
Ireland

1. Introduction

Congenital Diaphragmatic Hernia (CDH) is a severe and life threatening condition which can occur in isolation or with associated malformations. Congenital Heart Disease may be associated in up to 40% of cases with these infants often having a poor prognosis. This chapter aims to explore the association between CDH and congenital heart disease exploring the frequency of association, echocardiographic findings, prenatal diagnosis, use of cardiovascular biomarkers, surgical management and finally long term outcomes.

2. Methodology

Medline, PubMed, and Cochrane databases were searched for bibliography from Jan 1966 to December 2010. Key words used in the search were [Congenital Diaphragmatic Hernia], [Congenital heart disease], [Antenatal/Prenatal Diagnosis][Cardiovascular dysfunction], [Cardiac Biomarkers], [Surgical management and complications of CDH associated congenital heart disease], [Outcome in CDH associated congenital heart disease].

3. Frequency and type of congenital heart disease (CHD) associated with congenital diaphragmatic Hernia (CDH)

Congenital diaphragmatic Hernia (CDH) is a severe and life threatening malformation in infants. (Greenwood, Rosenthal et al. 1976) The reported incidence varies however the most recent series report a similar incidence of 1.4-4.5/10000 births (Dott, Wong et al. 2003) Infants with CDH may have an isolated diaphragmatic lesion, however complex CDH occurs with additional abnormalities either as part of a recognized syndrome, chromosomal abnormality or part of another major malformation accounts in 30 - 40% of cases. (Pober 2007) Associated malformations increase the mortality rate in infants with CDH. (Betremieux, Lionnais et al. 2002)

CDH may clinically mimic congenital heart disease, at birth with an infant who has low arterial oxygen saturations whom is difficult to oxygenate. In the largest multicentre cohort to date, Lin et al estimate the frequency of infants with non-syndromic CDH with associated congenital heart disease to vary from between 10–15% (Lin, Pober et al. 2007) The frequency of CDH and congenital heart disease rises to between 25-40% if infants with underlying syndromes and chromosomal abnormalities are included. (Lin, Pober et al. 2007) Harmath et al also found CDH was associated with cardiovascular anomalies in up to 43% of cases. (n=71)(Harmath, Hajdu et al. 2006)

Congenital heart Disease has prevalence in Europe of 7 per 1000 births. (Dolk, Loane et al.) The coexistence of CHD and congenital heart disease is often predictive of a poor prognosis (Sharland, Lockhart et al. 1992) Cohen et al reviewed 31 infants with CDH and congenital heart disease concluding that heart disease remains a significant risk factor for death in infants with CDH (Cohen, Rychik et al. 2002) The most frequent congenital heart defect associated with CDH was a Ventricular Septal Defect (VSD) (29%) which is also the most frequent congenital heart disease lesion in the paediatric population. This was followed by arch obstruction, hypoplastic left heart syndrome and Tetralogy of Fallot (13%). Their findings suggested that it was not the congenital heart lesion but severity of pulmonary hypoplasia that was the strongest predictor of poor outcome in this group. None of the infants with Tetralogy of Fallot or Transposition of the Great Arteries survived.(Cohen, Rychik et al. 2002) Similarly Dott et al found VSD to be the most commonly associated CHD lesion followed by atrial septal defect, coarctation of the aorta and hypoplastic left heart syndrome. (Dott, Wong et al. 2003)

Many congenital heart disease lesions for example, coarctation of the aorta, transposition of the great arteries, and truncus arteriosus are associated with an increased risk of pulmonary hypertension. This coupled with the existing risk of pulmonary hypertension in infants with CDH may account for the poor prognosis in this group. (Clarkson, Neutze et al. 1976; Levin, Mills et al. 1979; Kumar, Taylor et al. 1993; Sreeram, Petros et al. 1994)

Hypoplastic left heart syndrome (HLHS) is rarely associated with CDH (Nishimura, Taniguchi et al. 1992) despite many infants with CDH noted to have left heart hypoplasia. This is thought to result from compression by an enlarged right ventricle, but with structurally normal aortic and mitral valves and aortic arch with normal volume. (Lin, Pober et al. 2007)These infants are at increased risk of a low left ventricular mass which has been confirmed at post mortem.(Schwartz, Vermilion et al. 1994) Left ventricle mass measured on two-dimensional echocardiogram may predict outcome in infants with CDH, Schwartz et al concluded that left ventricular mass, indexed to patient weight was significantly diminished in patients with left sided CDH, (n=31) and this tool may be useful in determining suitability for Extracorporeal membrane oxygenation (ECMO) prior to surgical repair and possibly to help predict survival. (Schwartz, Vermilion et al. 1994) Case reports of infants with CDH and congenital heart disease exist with individual good outcomes. Noimark et al report a case of transposition of the great arteries VSD and CDH. The infant in their case survived, likely because the underlying cardiac defect could be repaired surgically.

4. Echocardiography in congenital diaphragmatic Hernia

Many studies have tried to correlate outcomes with the size of the main pulmonary artery (PA) measured by angiography or echocardiography. In infants with congenital heart disease indices of pulmonary artery size may be used to predict outcome before surgical correction of obstructive right heart lesions. (Suda, Bigras et al. 2000) These measures relate pulmonary artery size to the size of the aorta (McGoon Index) or body surface area (Nakta Index). Suda et al attempted to correlate the combined size of the proximal pulmonary arteries (as an indicator of pulmonary hypoplasia) with clinical outcome. They concluded that non survivors had significantly smaller hilar pulmonary arteries than survivors. (Suda, Bigras et al. 2000)

Similarly Okazaki et al reviewed the size of the left and right pulmonary arteries (LPA/RPA) on echocardiography to determine if pulmonary artery size and blood flow have prognostic value in CDH. (n=28) All patients who required treatment with Nitric Oxide (NO) had significantly smaller LPA and RPA and significantly smaller LPA/RPA ratio. All those died required treatment with NO (12%) and they concluded that a small LPA/RPA ratio appeared to be a simple highly reliable indicator of the necessity for NO therapy, and PA size may be a prognostic indicator in CDH. (Okazaki, Okawada et al. 2008)

Fetal echocardiographic measures of pulmonary hypoplasia and size in infants with CDH may be prognostic factors. (Thebaud, Azancot et al. 1997) Thebaud et at retrospectively measure the size of the cardiac ventricles, aorta and pulmonary arteries and calculated a measure of cardiac index comparing left and right ventricles and Aorta and pulmonary arteries. (n=32) Cardiac ventricular disproportion, expressed by the LV/RV ratio, appeared to correlate well with a poor outcome, concluding that Doppler flow studies may be helpful to improve understanding of left ventricular hypoplasia. (Thebaud, Azancot et al. 1997)

In the future methods such as tissue Doppler Imaging (TDI) may be useful as a prognostic indicator in CDH both pre and post surgery. In three cases TDI demonstrated improvement in both left and right sided myocardial performance index (MPI) following surgery, with both left and right MPI correlating well with clinical course. (Cua, Cooper et al. 2009)

5. Prenatal diagnosis of congenital heart disease associated with CDH - Planning for delivery

In the last twenty years prenatal diagnosis of CDH has improved significantly from 15% in the mid 1980s to almost 60% in the late 1990s. (Done, Gucciardo et al. 2008) Previously the outcome of fetuses with prenatally diagnosed CDH was thought to be poor, (Adzick, Vacanti et al. 1989) however as many cases are now diagnosed antenatally, prenatal diagnosis can no longer be considered a useful predictor of poor outcome.

CDH is suspected on antenatal ultrasound, in the presence of an absent or intrathoracic stomach bubble, cystic features noted in the chest, failure to identify the diaphragm, polyhyrdaminos, mediastinal and cardiac shift away from the side of the herniation and in extreme cases fatal hydrops. (Geary 1998) Polyhydraminos is found in more than 75% of pregnancies complicated by fetal CDH, and is thought to be a predictor of adverse outcome (Adzick, Harrison et al. 1985)

When CDH is suspected, associated anomalies must be looked for carefully on detailed fetal anomaly scans. As the association between chromosomal abnormalities and CDH is thought to range from 5% - 18% with many genetic disorders also being linked discussion should commence regarding fetal karyotyping (Cunniff, Jones et al. 1990; Bollmann, Kalache et al. 1995) The added incidence of chromosomal abnormalities, CDH and congenital heart disease, being as high as 25-40%,(Lin, Pober et al. 2007) favours karyotyping as a useful investigation.

Congenital heart disease is present in up to 15% of infants with CDH. (Pober 2007) These lesions may co exist because formation of the fetal diaphragm and the development of the fetal heart occur at similar times embryologically. (Noimark, Sellwood et al. 2000) Although the available data estimates antenatal diagnosis of congenital heart disease to be approximately 23%, this data is ten years old and when CDH is suspected, fetal echocardiography should be carried out by an experienced paediatric cardiologist. (Allan)

In the past it was suggested that left heart hypoplasia as detected on fatal echocardiogram may predict poor outcome.(Crawford, Drake et al. 1986; Sharland, Lockhart et al. 1992) In order to see if fetal echocardiographic variables could be used to predict outcome in fetuses with CDH, VanderWall et all reviewed echocardiographic evaluations in fetuses with CDH and compared them to normal fetuses. Left and right ventricular width were significantly less than controls of the same gestational age, as were the left ventricular volume and mass, however they concluded that no echocardiographic parameters could predict survival. (n=12) (VanderWall, Kohl et al. 1997) Fetal echocardiographic measures of pulmonary hypoplasia and size in infants with CDH may be prognostic factors. (Thebaud, Azancot et al. 1997) Thebaud et al retrospectively measured the size of the cardiac ventricles, aorta and pulmonary arteries and calculated these as a measure of cardiac index. (n=32) Cardiac ventricular disproportion, expressed by the LV/RV ratio, appeared to correlate well with a poor outcome, concluding that Doppler flow studies may be helpful to improve understanding of left ventricular hypoplasia. (Thebaud, Azancot et al. 1997) The pathophysiological process for the underdevelopment of the left side of the heart remains unclear, with mechanical compression from the herniated abdominal viscera still being the most likely cause, which is supported by the VanderWall findings. (Siebert, Haas et al. 1984; VanderWall, Kohl et al. 1997) I

Detecting CDH and congenital heart disease prenatally allows careful planning of both maternal and fetal care with multi speciality involvement. Delivery can be planned and should ideally take place in a tertiary referral centre with neonatal expertise available for elective intubation at birth and with easy access to paediatric surgery and paediatric cardiology if not available on site. In France in utero referral to a tertiary centre increased survival from 41-66%.(Gallot, Coste et al. 2006) The Canadian Neonatal Network demonstrated that centres receiving more than 12 infants per year with CDH had 13% higher survival rates. (Javid, Jaksic et al. 2004)

Prenatal diagnosis also allows early therapeutic decisions to be made. Recent evidence may favour the role of extra corporeal membrane oxygenation (ECMO). Infants who have antenatal measures of an abdnormal lung to head ratio for gestational age or herniation of the liver are more likely to require ECMO, therefore delivery should be planned in a tertiary centre who can provide ECMO. (Jani, Nicolaides et al. 2007). Other novel therapeutic measures include the use of Prostaglandin to maintain patency of the ductus arteriosus and to improve left ventricular diastolic dysfunction. (Inamura, Kubota et al. 2005)

Counselling should also be undertaken at this stage, as a number of children who survive CDH have higher indices of gastro oesophageal reflux, feeding dysfunction and bronchopulmonary dyplasia at one year of age. In the longer term those who survive CDH surgery have a significant risk of developmental delay and seizures. Prenatal diagnosis of CDH and congenital heart disease allows time for parental counselling, potential assessment of prognosis, planning for delivery in a Tertiary Referral centre and in the future may allow for antenatal intervention.

6. Use of cardiovascular biomarkers in children with CDH

Biochemical markers such a cardiac Troponin T and I and B-Type Natriuretic peptide (BNP), are well established markers of myocardial iscahemia and cardiac failure in adults and children (Koch and Singer 2003; Fromm 2007) (Spies, Haude et al. 1998)

BNP is a 32 amino acid ring structure which has its sequence present on chromosome 1. It is found in high concentration in the ventricles of the heart and is released in response to volume and pressure loading and ventricular stress. Pro BNP is the inactive precursor and is cleaved into BNP, the active component and N-terminal pro-BNP (NTpBNP), an inactive by-product. (El-Khuffash, Davis et al. 2008)BNP and NTpBNP levels are high at birth and fall slowly over the first two weeks of life. Normal ranges of BNP and NTpBNP have been established in neonates but vary depending on age of neonate and the testing kit used. (Ellis 1991) (Koch and Singer 2003) (El-Khuffash and Molloy 2009) (El-Khuffash and Molloy 2007)

BNP and NTpBNP are used to aid diagnosis, assess prognosis and to monitor ventricular dysfunction in various types of congenital heart disease. BNP is significantly increased in patients with ventricular dysfunction. (Koch, Zink et al. 2006) El Khuffash et al have also demonstrated the use of pro BNP and Troponin as an adjunct to echocardiography to predict poor neonatal outcome (grade III/IV intraventricular haemorrhage or death) in preterm infants with a PDA. (El-Khuffash, Slevin et al.)

Infants with persistent pulmonary hypertension of the newborn also have elevated levels of BNP (El-Khuffash and Molloy 2009) In the clinical setting, in the absence of paediatric cardiology onsite to confirm tricuspid regurgitation PPHN can be difficult to diagnose. This process may be aided using BNP, as BNP levels correlate well with pressure gradient across the tricuspid valve, and rising BNP levels indicate a worsening clinical condition (n=47). (Reynolds, Ellington et al. 2004) Pulmonary hypertension is a recognised complication of CDH. A small series (n=28) of infants with CDH showed that NTpBNP levels correlated well with estimated pulmonary artery pressure, Right Ventricle (RV) Tei index (a measure of global myocardial performance) and RV diastolic impairment. Infants with an elevated NTpBNP also had a worse prognosis. (Baptista, Rocha et al. 2008)

Troponins are the calcium binding site of the myofibrillary thin filament of the cardiac sacromere. There are three distinct proteins, Troponin T, Troponin C and Troponin I. The majority of cardiac troponins are bound in the contractile apparatus and Troponin C and I are released in response to myocardial ischaemia. Troponin T is a marker of cardiac injury in adults with ischaemic or haemorrhagic stroke in the absence of myocardial cell injury. (Fromm 2007)

Normal Troponin I levels in children are less than 2.0 ng/ml (n =120). (Hirsch, Landt et al. 1997) Fenton et al found increased Troponin I on admission in 57% of patients and at 12 hrs in 46% of pediatric intensive care patients admitted with septic shock and cardiovascular failure. (Fenton, Sable et al. 2004) Admission Troponin I levels inversely correlate with ejection fraction and fractional shortening and is directly proportional to wall stress. Children who had increased admission Troponin I had lower heart rate corrected mean velocity of circumferential fibre shortening (preload and heart rate independent measure of left ventricular systolic function) and higher wall stress (measure of afterload) compared with those with normal Troponin I. Admission Troponin I correlated with mortality. (Fenton, Sable et al. 2004) Troponin T is a good predictor of myocardial injury in asphyxiated neonates. (Hirsch, Landt et al. 1997) but has not yet been assessed in children with CDH.

7. Surgical management of CDH and congenital heart disease

Survival for infants with CDH has improved dramatically as new approaches to treatment arise. Gross first reported surgical repair of CDH in 1946. (Gross 1946) Since then the primary focus has shifted away from immediate surgery to stabilisation and optimising the physiological derangements in infants prior to surgery. (Chiu and Hedrick 2008). A better understanding of the underlying physiological processes that result from pulmonary hypoplasia has improved initial management and increased survival rates to as high as 90% in some tertiary paediatric centres over the last five years. (Boloker, Bateman et al. 2002; Downard and Wilson 2003; Chiu, Sauer et al. 2006)

Chiu et al found that the current focus of postnatal CDH management should be to firstly support oxygentation and ventilation while simultaneously trying to prevent ventilator induced lung damage, secondly to maintain cardiovascular stability though the use of ECMO, thirdly to treat pulmonary hypertension and finally to ultimately minimise overall morbidity. (Chiu and Hedrick 2008)In those with CDH surgical repair is no longer a surgical emergency, and mortality is not increased by waiting to improve ventilation.(Azarow, Messineo et al. 1997) (Langer, Filler et al. 1988) Those who undergo early versus late repair have similar survival rates (68% vs 62%) with the frequency of cardiac defects having the biggest influence on poor outcome, 26% in survivors vs 55% in non survivors. (n=111) (Rozmiarek, Qureshi et al. 2004) Infants are now managed with gentle ventilation strategies, which consist of permissive hypercapnea, that is accepting post ductal arterial pCO2 levels as high as 55 mmHg / 7.32 kPa with a compensated pH>7.35 provided cardiac performance and pulmonary pressures remain stable; preductal oxygen saturations >85% and restriction of airway pressure with early conversion to high-frequency oscillatory ventilation (HFOV) to minimise ventilator induced lung damage. (Chiu and Hedrick 2008) ECMO is now used to stabilise the infant with CDH, when the pulmonary vasculature is still reactive, however pulmonary hypertension and pulmonary hypoplasia remain the commonest causes of death in CDH infants while on ECMO. Many centres have suggested that survival has improved since the introduction of ECMO therapy however numbers are small. Patient selection for various treatments have not been standardised nor has criteria for separating patients with severe pulmonary hypoplasia, who have a high mortality from those with adequate lung development who have ductal shunting but whom have a lower mortality. (Azarow, Messineo et al. 1997)

In infants with CDH and congenital heart disease, surgery should be delayed until the pulmonary vascular resistance has decreased to acceptable levels. (Lin, Pober et al. 2007) The anatomic defect appears to be of secondary importance to the physiological effects of pulmonary hypoplasia. The spectrum of disorders associated with CDH such as pulmonary hypertension, left ventricular hypoplasia, ductal shunting still presents an overwhelming management challenge. A supra systemic elevation in the pulmonary vasculature resistance, that may coexist with both congenital heart disease and CDH produces a significant increase in the afterload on the right ventricle, having the potential to cause right ventricular failure, (Stayer and Liu) therefore medical management rather than surgical is important in the first instance. Providing the right ventricle with the means to 'pop off' through a shunt may prevent life threatening right heart failure. Maintaining the PDA serves this purpose as it remains patent through the presence of high flow in cases of suprasystemic RV pressure. If the PDA is restrictive, or closed intravenous prostaglandin may restore or maintain the patency of the PDA. (Bohn 2002; Berman Rosenzweig and Barst 2006)Pulmonary hypertension can be associated with both congenital heart malformations and CDH, with up to 34% of patients referred for evaluation of pulmonary hypertension in a tertiary centre having CDH. (Geggel 2004) It develops when the pulmonary vascular resistance (PVR) remains elevated after birth, resulting in left to right shunting through fetal circulatory pathways. (Stayer and Liu). Pulmonary hypertension in infants with congenital heart disease is most commonly seen in those who have a large left to right shunt. The size and location of the shunt as well as blood flow through the shunt are the most important risk factors for the development of pulmonary arterial hypertension. Infants with CDH have underdevelopment of the pulmonary vasculature, producing a fixed elevation of the PVR. Doppler echocardiography is necessary to measure the systolic tricuspid regurgitant jet in order to estimate pulmonary artery pressure. Treatment in infants with pulmonary hypertension depends on the underlying condition. Inhaled Nitric Oxide, a pulmonary vasodilator, has redefined the management of pulmonary hypertension, however to date no real benefit has been noted in those infants with congenital diaphragmatic hernia. (Shah, Jacob et al. 1994) (Stayer and Liu) (1997)

In the future intervention with fetal surgery may improve outcomes in children with CDH. Fetal surgery is justifiable if the natural history and pathophysiology of the disease are well understood, the prenatal diagnosis if accurate, if in utero correction is shown to be efficacious in animal models and if maternal risk is acceptably low. (Harrison and Adzick 1991)Percutaneous fetal valvuolplasty and atrial septostomy are exciting new advances in infants with critical aortic stenosis and hypoplastic left heart syndrome. (Allan)In infants with CDH there is a higher degree of pulmonary hypoplasia on the side of the lesion, fetal intervention may lead to sufficient parenchymal growth, by alleviating the space occupying lesion essentially formed by the abdominal viscera. (Deprest, Flake et al.; Gucciardo, Deprest et al. 2008) Measurements such as the lung-to-head ratio (LHR) and the position of the liver in utero (Jani, Keller et al. 2006) may help to predict the postnatal outcome for infants with isolated CDH, therefore helping to select those who may benefit from fetal intervention.

8. Long term outcomes in children with CDH and congenital heart disease

Throughout France, Australia and the United Kingdom survival rates of infants with isolated CDH are currently estimated to be between 50-70% with emphasis made on long term follow up.(Done, Gucciardo et al. 2008) As the survival rates continue to improve survivors are noted to have a higher incidence of respiratory, nutritional, musculoskeletal, neurological and gastrointestinal morbidities. (Chiu and Hedrick 2008) With newer treatments such as pre and post surgery ECMO survival rates of infants with CDH continue to improve. While ECMO may ultimately improve survival it is not without risk. Complications include perinatal asphyxia, hypoxaemia and intracranial bleeding secondary to the systemic heparinisation treatment used in conjunction with ECMO. (Frisk, Jakobson et al.) (Hedrick, Danzer et al. 2007)

Many studies to date focus on the short term neurodevelopmental outcomes of CDH survivors. Those infants who have not undergone ECMO as part of their treatment appear to have better outcomes than survivors who did receive ECMO. However these studies date back to the mid 1990s so further research is required. (Stolar, Crisafi et al. 1995) In the non ECMO therapy group, 8-9.5% are hearing impaired(Nobuhara, Lund et al. 1996), 8-13% have brain abnormalities(Lund, Mitchell et al. 1994) and up to 19% were developmentally delayed(Davenport, Rivlin et al. 1992). The long term survivors have lower intelligent quotient (IQ) with up to 50% experiencing emotional or behavioural problems. (Peetsold, Huisman et al. 2009)

There is a paucity of data on long term neurodevelopmental outcomes. Frisk et al followed a cohort of CDH survivors, (n=27) none of whom had undergone ECMO. Comparison to a peer control group revealed low rates of developmental issues reported in preschool infants, however as children progressed through school more educational difficulties became apparent. Between 23-46% of non-ECMO treated CDH survivors demonstrated clinically significant academic difficulties with parents reporting higher rates of attention difficulties and social problems. (Frisk, Jakobson et al.)

The Boston Circulatory Arrest trial provides the most comprehensive detail of neurodevelopmental outcomes in children following cardiac surgery. (Bellinger, Jonas et al. 1995; Bellinger, Wypij et al. 2003) Infants who had transposition of the great arteries who underwent the arterial switch operation were randomised to total circulatory arrest or low flow cardiopulmonary bypass during cardiac surgery and were followed up at eight years of age. Those who had longer postoperative stay in the cardiac intensive care unit had lower IQ scores at eight years of age. Use of circulatory arrest is associated with greater functional deficits than the use of low flow cardiopulmonary bypass, although both are associated with increased risk of neurodevelopmental problems. (Bellinger, Wypij et al. 2003) Children who undergo cardiac surgery for correction of congenital heart lesions also undergo circulatory arrest and this is associated with a higher risk of delayed motor development and neurological abnormalities at the age of one year than is surgery with low-flow bypass. Therefore infants who have CHD and an associated congenital heart defect will undergo a minimum of two surgeries and will have an increased risk of long term neurodevelopmental problems. Children who have congenital heart disease alone and who undergo surgery are at increased risk of growth and developmental problems as a result of cyanosis, heart failure, frequent hospitalisation, feeding difficulties and surgical intervention. This coupled with those surviving CDH surgery may contribute to the number of infants with short and long term neurodevelopmental problems.

9. Conclusion

CDH with associated congenital heart disease is a complex condition. With advances in both prenatal diagnosis and fetal surgical intervention these infants may have both better short and long term outcomes. Novel techniques such as the use of cardiovascular biomarkers may aid in the diagnosis of cardiovascular dysfunction, guide therapy and ultimately improve the outcomes in these infants.The paucity of data on long term cardiac function in infants surviving CDH surgery highlights an important area of future research.

10. References

Adzick, N. S., M. R. Harrison, et al. (1985). "Diaphragmatic hernia in the fetus: prenatal diagnosis and outcome in 94 cases." J Pediatr Surg 20 (4): 357-61.

Adzick, N. S., J. P. Vacanti, et al. (1989). "Fetal diaphragmatic hernia: ultrasound diagnosis and clinical outcome in 38 cases." J Pediatr Surg 24 (7): 654-7; discussion 657-8.

Allan, L. "Fetal cardiac scanning today." Prenat Diagn 30 (7): 639-43.

Azarow, K., A. Messineo, et al. (1997). "Congenital diaphragmatic hernia--a tale of two cities: the Toronto experience." J Pediatr Surg 32 (3): 395-400.

Baptista, M. J., G. Rocha, et al. (2008). "N-terminal-pro-B type natriuretic peptide as a useful tool to evaluate pulmonary hypertension and cardiac function in CDH infants." Neonatology 94 (1): 22-30.

Bellinger, D. C., R. A. Jonas, et al. (1995). "Developmental and neurologic status of children after heart surgery with hypothermic circulatory arrest or low-flow cardiopulmonary bypass." N Engl J Med 332 (9): 549-55.

Bellinger, D. C., D. Wypij, et al. (2003). "Neurodevelopmental status at eight years in children with dextro-transposition of the great arteries: the Boston Circulatory Arrest Trial." J Thorac Cardiovasc Surg 126 (5): 1385-96.

Berman Rosenzweig, E. and R. J. Barst (2006). "Pulmonary arterial hypertension : a comprehensive review of pharmacological treatment." Treat Respir Med 5 (2): 117-27.

Betremieux, P., S. Lionnais, et al. (2002). "Perinatal management and outcome of prenatally diagnosed congenital diaphragmatic hernia: a 1995-2000 series in Rennes University Hospital." Prenat Diagn 22 (11): 988-94.

Bohn, D. (2002). "Congenital diaphragmatic hernia." Am J Respir Crit Care Med 166 (7): 911-5.

Bollmann, R., K. Kalache, et al. (1995). "Associated malformations and chromosomal defects in congenital diaphragmatic hernia." Fetal Diagn Ther 10 (1): 52-9.

Boloker, J., D. A. Bateman, et al. (2002). "Congenital diaphragmatic hernia in 120 infants treated consecutively with permissive hypercapnea/spontaneous respiration/elective repair." J Pediatr Surg 37 (3): 357-66.

Chiu, P. and H. L. Hedrick (2008). "Postnatal management and long-term outcome for survivors with congenital diaphragmatic hernia." Prenat Diagn 28 (7): 592-603.

Chiu, P. P., C. Sauer, et al. (2006). "The price of success in the management of congenital diaphragmatic hernia: is improved survival accompanied by an increase in long-term morbidity?" J Pediatr Surg 41 (5): 888-92.

Clarkson, P. M., J. M. Neutze, et al. (1976). "The pulmonary vascular bed in patients with complete transposition of the great arteries." Circulation 53 (3): 539-43.

Cohen, M. S., J. Rychik, et al. (2002). "Influence of congenital heart disease on survival in children with congenital diaphragmatic hernia." J Pediatr 141 (1): 25-30.

Crawford, D. C., D. P. Drake, et al. (1986). "Prenatal diagnosis of reversible cardiac hypoplasia associated with congenital diaphragmatic hernia: implications for postnatal management." J Clin Ultrasound 14 (9): 718-21.

Cua, C. L., A. L. Cooper, et al. (2009). "Tissue Doppler changes in three neonates with congenital diaphragmatic hernia." Asaio J 55 (4): 417-9.

Cunniff, C., K. L. Jones, et al. (1990). "Patterns of malformation in children with congenital diaphragmatic defects." J Pediatr 116 (2): 258-61.

Davenport, M., E. Rivlin, et al. (1992). "Delayed surgery for congenital diaphragmatic hernia: neurodevelopmental outcome in later childhood." Arch Dis Child 67 (11): 1353-6.

Deprest, J. A., A. W. Flake, et al. "The making of fetal surgery." Prenat Diagn 30 (7): 653-67.

Dolk, H., M. Loane, et al. "Congenital heart defects in Europe: prevalence and perinatal mortality, 2000 to 2005." Circulation 123 (8): 841-9.

Done, E., L. Gucciardo, et al. (2008). "Prenatal diagnosis, prediction of outcome and in utero therapy of isolated congenital diaphragmatic hernia." Prenat Diagn 28 (7): 581-91.

Dott, M. M., L. Y. Wong, et al. (2003). "Population-based study of congenital diaphragmatic hernia: risk factors and survival in Metropolitan Atlanta, 1968-1999." Birth Defects Res A Clin Mol Teratol 67 (4): 261-7.

Downard, C. D. and J. M. Wilson (2003). "Current therapy of infants with congenital diaphragmatic hernia." Semin Neonatol 8 (3): 215-21.

El-Khuffash, A., P. G. Davis, et al. (2008). "Cardiac troponin T and N-terminal-pro-B type natriuretic peptide reflect myocardial function in preterm infants." J Perinatol 28 (7): 482-6.

El-Khuffash, A. and E. Molloy (2009). "The Use of N-Terminal-Pro-BNP in Preterm Infants." Int J Pediatr 2009 : 175216.

El-Khuffash, A. and E. J. Molloy (2007). "Are B-type natriuretic peptide (BNP) and N-terminal-pro-BNP useful in neonates?" Arch Dis Child Fetal Neonatal Ed 92 (4): F320-4.

El-Khuffash, A. F., M. Slevin, et al. "Troponin T, N-terminal pro natriuretic peptide and a patent ductus arteriosus scoring system predict death before discharge or neurodevelopmental outcome at 2 years in preterm infants." Arch Dis Child Fetal Neonatal Ed .

Ellis, A. K. (1991). "Serum protein measurements and the diagnosis of acute myocardial infarction." Circulation 83 (3): 1107-9.

Fenton, K. E., C. A. Sable, et al. (2004). "Increases in serum levels of troponin I are associated with cardiac dysfunction and disease severity in pediatric patients with septic shock." Pediatr Crit Care Med 5 (6): 533-8.

Frisk, V., L. S. Jakobson, et al. "Long-term neurodevelopmental outcomes of congenital diaphragmatic hernia survivors not treated with extracorporeal membrane oxygenation." J Pediatr Surg 46 (7): 1309-18.

Fromm, R. E., Jr. (2007). "Cardiac troponins in the intensive care unit: common causes of increased levels and interpretation." Crit Care Med 35 (2): 584-8.

Gallot, D., K. Coste, et al. (2006). "Antenatal detection and impact on outcome of congenital diaphragmatic hernia: a 12-year experience in Auvergne, France." Eur J Obstet Gynecol Reprod Biol 125 (2): 202-5.

Geary, M. (1998). "Management of congenital diaphragmatic hernia diagnosed prenatally: an update." Prenat Diagn 18 (11): 1155-8.

Geggel, R. L. (2004). "Conditions leading to pediatric cardiology consultation in a tertiary academic hospital." Pediatrics 114 (4): e409-17.

Greenwood, R. D., A. Rosenthal, et al. (1976). "Cardiovascular abnormalities associated with congenital diaphragmatic hernia." Pediatrics 57 (1): 92-7.

Gross, R. E. (1946). "Congenital hernia of the diaphragm." Am J Dis Child 71 : 579-92.

Gucciardo, L., J. Deprest, et al. (2008). "Prediction of outcome in isolated congenital diaphragmatic hernia and its consequences for fetal therapy." Best Pract Res Clin Obstet Gynaecol 22 (1): 123-38.

Harmath, A., J. Hajdu, et al. (2006). "Associated malformations in congenital diaphragmatic hernia cases in the last 15 years in a tertiary referral institute." Am J Med Genet A 140 (21): 2298-304.

Harrison, M. R. and N. S. Adzick (1991). "The fetus as a patient. Surgical considerations." Ann Surg 213 (4): 279-91; discussion 277-8.

Hedrick, H. L., E. Danzer, et al. (2007). "Liver position and lung-to-head ratio for prediction of extracorporeal membrane oxygenation and survival in isolated left congenital diaphragmatic hernia." Am J Obstet Gynecol 197 (4): 422 e1-4.

Hirsch, R., Y. Landt, et al. (1997). "Cardiac troponin I in pediatrics: normal values and potential use in the assessment of cardiac injury." J Pediatr 130 (6): 872-7.

Inamura, N., A. Kubota, et al. (2005). "A proposal of new therapeutic strategy for antenatally diagnosed congenital diaphragmatic hernia." J Pediatr Surg 40 (8): 1315-9.

Jani, J., R. L. Keller, et al. (2006). "Prenatal prediction of survival in isolated left-sided diaphragmatic hernia." Ultrasound Obstet Gynecol 27 (1): 18-22.

Jani, J., K. H. Nicolaides, et al. (2007). "Observed to expected lung area to head circumference ratio in the prediction of survival in fetuses with isolated diaphragmatic hernia." Ultrasound Obstet Gynecol 30 (1): 67-71.

Javid, P. J., T. Jaksic, et al. (2004). "Survival rate in congenital diaphragmatic hernia: the experience of the Canadian Neonatal Network." J Pediatr Surg 39 (5): 657-60.

Koch, A. and H. Singer (2003). "Normal values of B type natriuretic peptide in infants, children, and adolescents." Heart 89 (8): 875-8.

Koch, A., S. Zink, et al. (2006). "B-type natriuretic peptide in paediatric patients with congenital heart disease." Eur Heart J 27 (7): 861-6.

Kumar, A., G. P. Taylor, et al. (1993). "Pulmonary vascular disease in neonates with transposition of the great arteries and intact ventricular septum." Br Heart J 69 (5): 442-5.

Langer, J. C., R. M. Filler, et al. (1988). "Timing of surgery for congenital diaphragmatic hernia: is emergency operation necessary?" J Pediatr Surg 23 (8): 731-4.

Levin, D. L., L. J. Mills, et al. (1979). "Morphologic development of the pulmonary vascular bed in experimental coarctation of the aorta." Circulation 60 (2): 349-54.

Lin, A. E., B. R. Pober, et al. (2007). "Congenital diaphragmatic hernia and associated cardiovascular malformations: type, frequency, and impact on management." Am J Med Genet C Semin Med Genet 145C (2): 201-16.

Lund, D. P., J. Mitchell, et al. (1994). "Congenital diaphragmatic hernia: the hidden morbidity." J Pediatr Surg 29 (2): 258-62; discussion 262-4.

Nishimura, M., A. Taniguchi, et al. (1992). "Hypoplastic left heart syndrome associated with congenital right-sided diaphragmatic hernia and omphalocele." Chest 101 (1): 263-4.

Nobuhara, K. K., D. P. Lund, et al. (1996). "Long-term outlook for survivors of congenital diaphragmatic hernia." Clin Perinatol 23 (4): 873-87.

Noimark, L., M. Sellwood, et al. (2000). "Transposition of the great arteries, ventricular septal defect and diaphragmatic hernia in a fetus: the role of prenatal diagnosis in helping to predict postnatal survival." Prenat Diagn 20 (11): 924-6.

Okazaki, T., M. Okawada, et al. (2008). "Significance of pulmonary artery size and blood flow as a predictor of outcome in congenital diaphragmatic hernia." Pediatr Surg Int 24 (12): 1369-73.

Peetsold, M. G., J. Huisman, et al. (2009). "Psychological outcome and quality of life in children born with congenital diaphragmatic hernia." Arch Dis Child 94 (11): 834-40.

Pober, B. R. (2007). "Overview of epidemiology, genetics, birth defects, and chromosome abnormalities associated with CDH." Am J Med Genet C Semin Med Genet 145C (2): 158-71.

Reynolds, E. W., J. G. Ellington, et al. (2004). "Brain-type natriuretic peptide in the diagnosis and management of persistent pulmonary hypertension of the newborn." Pediatrics 114 (5): 1297-304.

Rozmiarek, A. J., F. G. Qureshi, et al. (2004). "Factors influencing survival in newborns with congenital diaphragmatic hernia: the relative role of timing of surgery." J Pediatr Surg 39 (6): 821-4; discussion 821-4.

Schwartz, S. M., R. P. Vermilion, et al. (1994). "Evaluation of left ventricular mass in children with left-sided congenital diaphragmatic hernia." J Pediatr 125 (3): 447-51.

Shah, N., T. Jacob, et al. (1994). "Inhaled nitric oxide in congenital diaphragmatic hernia." J Pediatr Surg 29 (8): 1010-4; discussion 1014-5.

Sharland, G. K., S. M. Lockhart, et al. (1992). "Prognosis in fetal diaphragmatic hernia." Am J Obstet Gynecol 166 (1 Pt 1): 9-13.

Siebert, J. R., J. E. Haas, et al. (1984). "Left ventricular hypoplasia in congenital diaphragmatic hernia." J Pediatr Surg 19 (5): 567-71.

Spies, C., V. Haude, et al. (1998). "Serum cardiac troponin T as a prognostic marker in early sepsis." Chest 113 (4): 1055-63.

Sreeram, N., A. Petros, et al. (1994). "Progressive pulmonary hypertension after the arterial switch procedure." Am J Cardiol 73 (8): 620-1.

Stayer, S. A. and Y. Liu "Pulmonary hypertension of the newborn." Best Pract Res Clin Anaesthesiol 24 (3): 375-86.

Stolar, C. J., M. A. Crisafi, et al. (1995). "Neurocognitive outcome for neonates treated with extracorporeal membrane oxygenation: are infants with congenital diaphragmatic hernia different?" J Pediatr Surg 30 (2): 366-71; discussion 371-2.

Suda, K., J. L. Bigras, et al. (2000). "Echocardiographic predictors of outcome in newborns with congenital diaphragmatic hernia." Pediatrics 105 (5): 1106-9.

Thebaud, B., A. Azancot, et al. (1997). "Congenital diaphragmatic hernia: antenatal prognostic factors. Does cardiac ventricular disproportion in utero predict outcome and pulmonary hypoplasia?" Intensive Care Med 23 (10): 10062-9.

VanderWall, K. J., T. Kohl, et al. (1997). "Fetal diaphragmatic hernia: echocardiography and clinical outcome." J Pediatr Surg 32 (2): 223-5; discussion 225-6.

(1997). "Inhaled nitric oxide and hypoxic respiratory failure in infants with congenital diaphragmatic hernia. The Neonatal Inhaled Nitric Oxide Study Group (NINOS)." Pediatrics 99 (6): 838-45.

9

Congenital Diaphragmatic Hernia: State of the Art Reconstruction- Biologics Versus Synthetics

Anne C. Fischer
UT Southwestern Medical School &
Dallas Children's Medical Center
USA

1. Introduction

1.1 Impact of therapeutics on survival

Survival rates to hospital discharge for a neonate with a diagnosis of congenital diaphragmatic hernia (CDH) appear to have improved remarkably when comparing reports of 82-93% survival out of single institutions to the overall survival rate of 69% from tertiary centers in the Congenital Diaphragmatic Hernia Study Group (CDHSG). Others continue to dispute such outstanding gains, attributing them both to patient recruitment and a case selection bias at tertiary referral centers (Stege et al., 2004). In contrast, significantly lower survival rates of 54-56% have been reported from population-based studies in the UK and Australia despite their implementation of the same strategy of presurgical stabilization, permissive hypercapnea and gentilation with high frequency ventilator modes (Levison, 2006). Population based studies typically include more nonsurvivors than tertiary referral centers who capture only those who survived to arrival the other caveat is how to best track all those diagnosed prenatally.

The UK and Australian experience was similarly reflected in a US population-based study using the KIDS' Inpatient Database, in which overall survival was 66% (Sola et al., 2010). Strikingly, the postoperative survival in the KIDS' Database was much higher at 86% which reflects the degree of case selection bias involved in those offered surgical repair. This discordance supports those who argue the higher survival reports out of single institutions often reflect an underlying unintended case selection bias. Despite all the advances in intensive care management of diaphragmatic hernias and ventilation of critically ill neonates, there remains a >35% of live-born infants with a CDH who do not survive to transport, making the diagnosis of CDH accountable for >1% of all annual infant mortality (Clark et al., 1998) and the highest in-hospital neonatal mortality of all birth defects (CDC, 2007).

Clearly a subset of children with CDH remains predisposed to fatality despite the availability of novel therapies. Thus being able to predict which subset is most likely to benefit from experimental or more aggressive therapies, as well as the consideration of withdrawal of care when suitable, would be remarkably useful to best target novel therapeutics for best benefit. In fact now there are many novel therapies directed at the high risk subset and liberally utilized given the inability to risk stratify patients. These novel therapeutics include the selective use of ECMO (Khan & Lally, 2005), pulmonary vasodilators such as inhaled nitric oxide (Okuyama et al., 2002; Finer & Barrington, 2001), and sildenafil (Hunter et al., 2009), permissive hypercapnea and high frequency oscillatory ventilation (Miguet et al., 1995), treatment at high volume centers (Stege et al., 2004), fetal surgery/ tracheal occlusion without proven survival advantage (Harrison et al., 2003), and the futuristic application of partial liquid ventilation (Hirschl, 2004). Other therapies often utilized, such as the use of exogenous surfactant, have not been shown to improve survival rates in the premature infant with CDH; although, they have not been analyzed in a randomized control trial to fully prove efficacy (Lally et al., 2004).

2. Defect size: Prognostic relevance

The coexistence of marked pulmonary hypertension and pulmonary hypoplasia are the key factors identifying the subset of infants that are more likely to die or survive with significant morbidity. The ability to identify prenatally those with problematic pulmonary hypertension and hypoplasia has not yet been realized. There are many indirect metrics for prenatal predictors of mortality which at best can estimate postnatal outcomes with variable accuracy. Those prenatal predictors of mortality include fetal liver position (Kunisaki et al., 2008; Kitano et al. 2005; Hedrick et al., 2007), fetal lung volumes (Nishie et al., 2009) and lung area-to-head ratios (LHR) (Bretelle et al., 2007; Deprest et al., 2009). Notably all of these measures are proxies for the severity of underlying pulmonary hypoplasia secondary to the degree of visceral herniation. In an isolated left CDH, liver position is the best prenatal predictor of outcome. In those with liver up, ECMO was required in 80% of fetuses compared to 25% for those with liver down: survival rate was 45% for the liver up subset, compared to 93% for those with liver down (Hedrick et al., 2007). In similar fashion, a low LHR (<1.0) predicted an increased incidence of ECMO (75%) with a lower survival rate (35%) (Hedrick et al., 2007), but the LHR was not useful in those <24 weeks GA (Yang et al, 2007). There are other factors used to predict survival which include birth weight >2.5 Kg (Casaccia et al., 2006), and coexistence of chromosomal and cardiac anomalies (Graziano et al., 2006; Witters et al., 2001; Hilfiker et al., 1998). The most common chromosomal anomalies identified in CDH were trisomies 13, 18, and 21, the most common syndrome was Fryns syndrome, and either a hypoplastic left heart syndrome, coarctation of the aorta, or tetralogy of fallot for the complex heart disease identified.

The size of the defect is the best corollary for the degree of pulmonary hypoplasia. *In vivo* CDH animal models have demonstrated the association between varying the size of the defect and the resultant degree of pulmonary hypoplasia in both lambs and toxicological rodent models, where the gestational timing of the insult is the factor determining defect size and outcome (Hilfiker et al., 1998). The CDHSG identified the size of the diaphragmatic hernia defect as the major factor influencing outcome based on a 9 year multi-institutional registry of 3062 CDH patients (Lally et al., 2007). Notably those with a primary repair had a 95% survival rate compared to those requiring a patch repair at 79%

in contrast to an overall survival rate of 69% for all comers. Thus a patch repair has become synonymous with larger defect sizes. Among those requiring a patch repair, those with the largest defect possible - diaphragm agenesis, had the worst odds of survival at 57% with an odds ratio of 14.04 times the mortality of those who underwent a primary repair (Singh et al., 1999). Neonates with a diaphragm agenesis are well known to be associated with a high mortality (Brindle et al., 2011).

The significance of the diaphragm defect was confirmed by the Canadian Pediatric Surgery Network (CAPSNet) in a 5-year 212 patient database which showed that a patch repair was the only significant predictor of mortality with an odds ratio of 17:1 (Skargard et al., 2005). Those requiring patch repairs were independently associated with secondary morbidities such as the number of ventilator days and the need for oxygen at discharge. The Canadian study was illustrative given the absence of other confounding variables to which to attribute the mortality risk. The subset requiring a patch repair did not also have a higher incidence of other risk variables such as birth weight, gestational age, or the presence of cardiac or chromosomal anomalies. Instead in CAPSNet, those requiring a patch repair differed from those not requiring a patch repair strictly only by their need for ECMO and SNAP-II score, both measures of disease severity. The SNAP-II score, the score for neonatal acute physiology, is a well described and validated metric for the predictor of mortality in CDH. Thus the need for a patch repair is our best proxy for defect size, and by showing a higher mortality risk associated with patch repair , defect size is the best surrogate marker for the severity of pulmonary hypoplasia.

The spectrum of defect sizes parallels the prenatal timing of initial detection prenatally and the underlying degree of associated pulmonary hypoplasia. Prenatally the degree of visceral herniation has been a good proxy for the size of the defect: the grade of herniation of the stomach into the chest (Kitano et al., 2011), herniation of the liver into the chest (Mullassery et al., 2010), herniation of the liver combined with the LHR for prediction of ECMO usage and mortality (Hedrick et al., 2007). All these prenatal measurements are used as predictors of outcome and are the best proxies for the size of the defect and the severity of underlying pulmonary hypertension. The converse is also true that there is a subset of left sided CDH neonates who have no evidence of visceral herniation *in utero* and have a remarkably higher survival rate, lower prosthetic graft rate, and lower ECMO utilization compared to the control group (Valfre et al., 2011). This finding documented what was well recognized clinically - that the presentation of a CDH postnatally is associated with smaller defects, a lower need for prosthetic graft repairs than those who present early in gestation, and better outcomes. To date the actual defect size remains immeasurable by prenatal or postnatal imaging. Although defect size is singularly predictive of outcome in both overall survival (Singh et al.,1999; Skargard et al., 2005) and longterm morbidities (Raval et al., 2011), such as gastroesophageal reflux, altered pulmonary function and poor auxological outcomes, a numeric value for the defect size has not been accurately recorded in most studies or tracked in registries. Similarly there is no identified cut-off value that defines the large defects or agenesis. Efforts continue to focus ideally on attempting to determine defect size prenatally or preoperatively to risk stratify patients and better match high risk patients with high risk therapies, with improved counseling and avoiding risky therapies in low risk patients.

3. Patch repairs: Synthetics versus Biologics

3.1 Primary repair

Primary repair is the desired standard for the closure of the diaphragmatic defect. Due to all the advances above, the cohort of more complicated repairs is increasing and long term follow up is available on the durability of various types of repair. In all cases, closure needs to ensure durability to best avoid re-herniation since re-operative surgery is not trivial in these children. The percentage of neonates undergoing repair is not clear, since different centers vary as to patient recruitment and which patients are deemed unsalvageable for surgical intervention. Not all such patients are included in registries. For an approximate estimate of the percentage repaired, analysis of the KIDS' Inpatient Database limited to all patients less than 8 days of age admitted to any hospital with a diagnosis of CDH identified 2774 patients, of which only 1095 underwent operative repair (Sola et al., 2010). Thus approximately a third of all neonates with a CDH are offered surgical repair. This analysis that a third were actually offered surgical repair was confirmed by a different KIDS' Database analysis (Raval et al., 2011). Thus not all CDH neonates are offered repair, which implies those that are offered repair represent a case selection bias. In contrast, the CDHSG registry with 3062 live born CDH infants from tertiary institutions reported a larger percentage of up to 82.4% of those tracked in the registry were surgically repaired: 43% had a primary repair, 22.1% had a patch repair and 15% had complete agenesis (Singh et al., 2009).

3.2 Synthetic and biologics

Given the expected variations of surgical preference in determining whether a patch is used, there is a trend to liberally use patches to avoid tension and compartment syndromes (Loff et al., 2005; Bax and Collins, 1984). So some elect patch repair to improve physiologic results and others use patches only when primary repair cannot be physically achieved. Current practice is to create a tension-free closure such that prosthetic patches are used only when a defect is not amenable to a primary repair, after mobilizing the posterior diaphragmatic leaf, or as in cases of agenesis. The most common material used in prosthetic patches is polytetrafluoroethylene (PTFE: Gore-tex® [WL Gore and Associates, Flagstaff, AZ]); other prosthetic materials have included composite grafts with Goretex®, SILAS-TIC© (Dow Corning, Midland, MI), Dacron, polypropylene and fluorinated polyester but none of these have been used as frequently as Gore-Tex. The concern with prosthetics is their inability to accommodate thoracic growth leading to chest restriction, chest wall deformity (Greig & Azmy, 1990), and reherniation (Hajer et al., 1998). PTFE induces no tissue ingrowth and incites a high inflammatory response with essentially no biologic fusion to the surrounding diaphragmatic muscle.

Numerous biologics have been applied to CDH defects to create a lattice, allowing for tissue ingrowth of autologous tissue (see Table 1). Biologics ideally, with tissue incorporation, would be able to avoid the reherniation rates characteristic of prosthetic patches and the scoliosis from the inability of a prosthetic to compensate for age-related growth of the thoracic cavity. The most commonly used acellular bioprosthetic patches include Surgisis-Gold (Cook Biotech, Lafayette, IN), Permacol (Tissue Science Laboratories Inc, Andover, Mass), Alloderm (LifeCell Inc, Branchburg, NJ), or recent composites with a synthetic sandwiched as an overlay to a bioprosthetic, such as Gore-tex® and Surgisis®(See Figure

1D) Prior bilayer patches incorporated both Gore-tex® and Marlex® which demonstrated only one recurrence (3.5%) (Riehle et al., 2007) which suggested a benefit of sandwiching a synthetic with a monofilament mesh to induce tissue incorporation.

Bioprosthetic	Source	Matrix	Company
Surgisis	**Porcine**	Non-crosslinked acellular small intestinal submucosa 8-ply	Cook biotech, west lafayette, ind
Permacol	**Porcine**	Chemically cross-linked acellular dermal collagen	Tissue science laboratories, ndover, mass.
Alloderm	**Human**	Non-crosslinked acellular dermal matrix	Lifecell, inc. branchburg nj
Peri-guard	**Bovine**	Chemically cross-linked pericardium	Synovis surgical innovations, st paul, minn
Veritas	**Bovine**	Non-crosslinked pericardium	Synovis surgical innovations, st paul, minn

Table 1. Types of bioprosthetic materials for grafts

Synthetic patch repairs emerged historically as the predominant method of tension-free closure of defects not amenable to primary repair (Levison et al., 2006). Despite three decades of experience with synthetic patches, which offer a superb short term solution, recurrence rates are reported as high as 41% -46% at a median follow up of 12 months (Moss et al., 2001; Jancelewicz et al., 2010), compared to 10-22% rate following primary closure in long-term survivors (Jancelewicz et al., 2010; Cohen & Reid, 1981). Long-term studies showed that prosthetic grafts can result in recurrences in up to 50% of patients by 3 years of age (Moss et al., 2001). The risk factors associated with an increased risk of recurrence in graft repairs include all factors discussed earlier that are associated with a worse disease severity, such as right side CDH laterality, ECMO therapy, size and need for a patch (Hajer et al., 1998).

Only the history of a patch repair was independently predictive of a subsequent diaphragmatic hernia recurrence when compared to multiple prenatal markers of CDH severity in a multivariant regression analysis (Jancelewicz et al., 2010). The higher rates of recurrence in synthetic patch repairs are thought to be secondary to a lack of tissue incorporation and inability to accommodate growth, so that tension over time causes the patches to separate from the thoracic wall as well as lead to chest wall deformities. Notably there is an increased prevalence of chest deformities in 50% of patients by 3 years of age, equivalent to the incidence of recurrences (Vanamo et al., 1996). In fact there is a bimodal distribution of recurrences with Gore-Tex®: an early peak at 2 months and a later peak at 20 months (Moss et al., 2001). This bimodal distribution of graft failure has been confirmed in other studies (Mitchell et al., 2008).

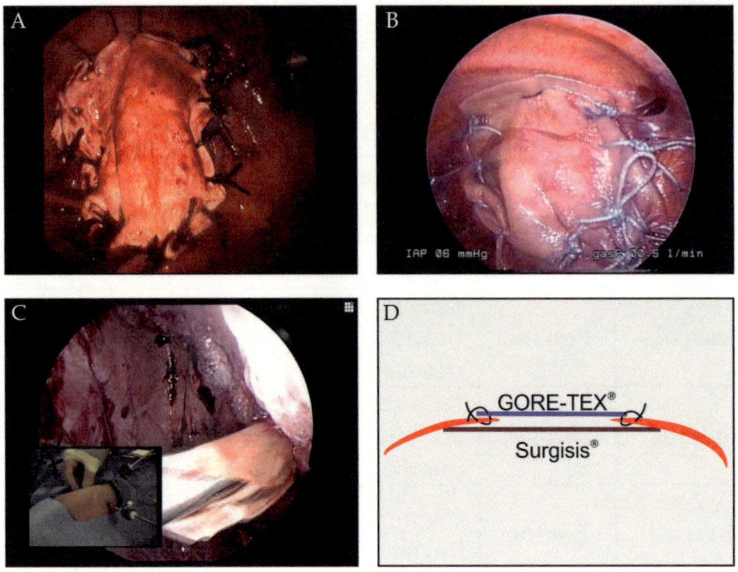

Fig. 1. Comparison of Gore-tex® and Surgisis®. A. Gortex patch sewn in situ, B. Thoracoscopic view of Surgisis® patch in situ. C. Technique of thoroscopically introducing a patch, D. A modified patch combining Gore-Tex (nonabsorbable mesh) and Surgisis (biodegradable prosthetic material) as a bilayer composite graft. (Courtesy of Dr. Mark Wulkan at Emory University School of Medicine & Emory Children's Center)

Bioprosthetics have been widely applied and successful in a variety of hernia repairs and closures of abdominal wall defects. They provide a temporary acellular scaffold that supports native tissue ingrowth and ability to accommodate growth. Since these bioprosthetics are acellular, they are nonimmunogenic. Given the high recurrence rates associated with Gore-Tex®, one study compared Surgisis® (a 4- or 8- ply porcine-derived extracellular matrix from small intestine submucosa) to Gore-Tex® in 72 newborns, reporting no significant difference in recurrence rates (38% and 44%, respectively: Grethel EJ et al., 2006). Graft failures occurred early with 92% of Surgisis® failures and 75% of Gore-Tex® failures within 1 year. A Surgisis® repair was associated with higher frequency of operative bowel obstruction, (Jancelewicz et al., 2010; St. Peter SD et al., 2007) and was possibly proinflammatory (Baroncello JB et al., 2008). In a recent *in vivo* porcine model, Surgisis® resulted in better tissue integration than PTFE, enhanced incorporation of skeletal muscle in replacement of the acellular graft with higher collagen-forming fibroblasts, and lower fibrotic reaction (Gonzalez et al., 2011). In contrast, PTFE induced a thick fibrotic capsule consistent with an inflammatory reaction that exceeded that of Surgisis®. Perforated and 8-ply Surgisis® is currently being trialed in composite grafts with Gore-Tex® (Fig 1). Remodeling of collagen-based patches in CDH applications has been analyzed in animal models to compare Surgisis®, a porcine intestinal submucosa to Gore-Tex® (Lantis et al., 2000). The collagen-based repairs showed more integration, increased vascularization, fibroblastic ingrowth, and less inflammation compared to the high inflammatory reaction at the PTFE-diaphragmatic interface. This proinflammatory reaction along the synthetic to diaphragm interface may explain the recurrence rates seen.

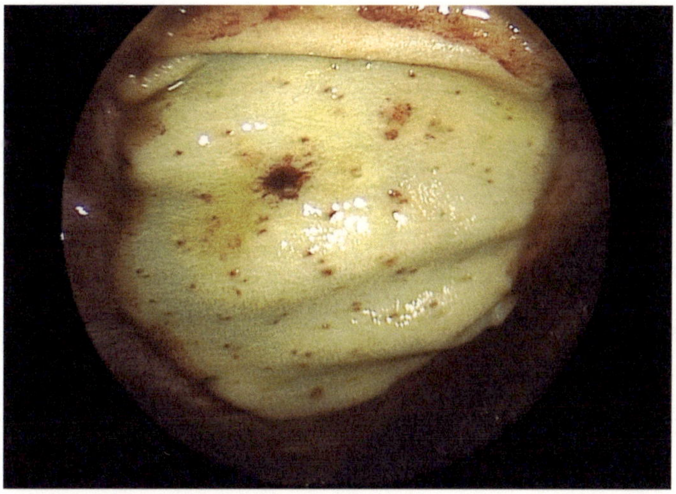

Thoroscopic view of a Permacol Patch in CDH repair.

Fig. 2. Intrathoroscopic Visualization of a Permacol® patch used in a neonatal CDH repair 2 months after placement to show tissue incorporation

Permacol®, less widely used in CDH applications but popularized in adults, is an extracelluar matrix of chemically crosslinked porcine dermal collagen. In a case report of abdominovisceral disproportion and a retrospective CDH series, Permacol® demonstrated durability with no recurrences in a median follow up of 20 months, the time frame in which Gore-Tex® demonstrated a 28% failure rate (Richards et al., 2005; Mitchell et al., 2008). The type of tissue incorporation with Permacol® is illustrated in Figure 2 above, in a baby 2 months following a CDH repair with Permacol. This is an intrathoroscopic caudal view at the diaphragm due a second surgery for a previously unrecognized lung anomaly; no suture line is evident here which is so evident with the use of a synthetic. Also there are multiple areas of tissue ingrowth from the side of the Permacol against the liver (note red punctate areas as islands of tissue ingrowth). The cross-linking of lysine and hydroxylysine residues within the collagen fibers of Permacol® imparts a higher resistance to collagenases and improved durability compared to other bioprosthetics (Richards, et al. 2005).

Composite patch repairs, such as Gore-Tex®/Marlex synthetic patches, have been reported used in humans with only a 3% recurrence rate, followed for a median of 47 months, but had an unusual comorbidity of a 17% splenectomy rate which is nontrivial in this population (Riehle et al., 2007). The search for an ideal material for CDH repairs is an ongoing active area of investigation. Clearly controlled trials are needed to compare the outcomes from composite grafts (such as Gore-Tex® with a bioprosthetic) to other bioprosthetics and synthetics; likewise bioengineered grafts are potentially promising.

3.3 Autologous grafts

Autologous tissue is often limited in size and viability in a neonate, as well as problematic given the heparinization needed for possible ECMO. Often autologous tissue is not ideal for initial repair. Thus, autologous tissue is used for more often in the setting of staged repair, recurrent reherniation or when a child is older and the tissue is more robust or of sufficient size. The first patch repair described for a CDH repair used autologous tissue and a split abdominal wall muscle flap (Simpson & Gossage, 1971). The split abdominal wall muscle flap was idealized to place a *vascularized* and *innervated* tissue flap repair that will both accommodate growth and cover a large diaphragmatic defect. This flap has not been popularized and thus remains as infrequently used option. A single institution series retrospectively reviewed their use: in 13 patients, 5 of which were done on ECMO, there were no recurrences in 6 years excluding the one patient dying in the ECMO subset from right heart failure (Brant- Zawadzki et al., 2007). The muscle flap has yet to gain widespread acceptance as a first- line procedure (Nasr et al., 2010) and is often reserved for an older child with greater muscle capacity and robustness (Masumoto et al., 2007).

Type of graft	Pros	Cons	Citations
Anterior abdominal wall muscle flap	Primary repair	Abdominal bulge	Nasr 2010, Scaife 2008, Simpson & Gossage, 1971
Reversed latissimus dorsi muscle	Innervated, wide flap	Staged repair	Sydorak 2003
Free fascia lata repair	Strongest fascia	Loss of extremity function @ harvest site, hematoma	Sugiyama 2011, Clark 1998

Table 2. Autologous muscle or fascial flaps

Other autologous grafts are utilized for the repair of the recurrent CDH and include the reversed latissimus dorsi muscle flap (Sydorak et al., 2003); and the free fascia lata repair (Sugiyama et al., 2011). The reversed latissimus dorsi muscle flap is both vascularized and innervated and has shown promise in 7 patients with no reherniation in a medium follow up of 24 months (Sydorak et al., 2003). This use of autologous tissue is best utilized for the repair of recurrences, and allows not only a pleuroperitoneal separation, but also a potentially functional diaphragmatic reconstruction: this later point needs to be proven in longterm studies given the neural anastomosis. The free fascia lata graft has the potential of using the strongest fascia but may result in loss of extremity function, is not innervated, and its application in children or neonates is not well popularized. All autologous tissue repairs can be problematic if utilized in the setting of a heparinized circuit such as ECMO, particularly with a large surface area of dissection with associated tissue edema. All of these autologous grafts are cautioned to be used with a liberal application of a staged abdominal wall closure, particularly in those on ECMO support with resultant significant tissue edema.

4. Impact of minimally invasive surgery on recurrences

The revolution in minimally invasive surgery (MIS) naturally allowed the application of MIS to the repair of CDH patients. Theoretically, a minimally invasive repair would minimize the deleterious effects of open surgery while being able to decompress the CDH lung. Many reports have proclaimed the feasibility and initial safety of MIS in its application to CDH repairs (Yang et al., 2005; Shah et al., 2009).

Since the technique is relatively new, there was a careful case selection bias in order to select those patients most suitable. Despite a case selection bias, there is already a significant incidence of recurrences in those repaired by MIS, as opposed to those undergoing an open repair, when examining 151 MIS repairs in the CDH registry out of a total of 4516 patients repaired (Tsao & Lally et al., 2011). Case selection was intended and evident in the disparate use of ECMO (Cho et al., 2009) and targeting groups with favorable criteria such as ventilator stability and absence of stomach or liver herniation (Yang et al., 2005; Kim et al., 2009). Thus, the higher in-hospital recurrence rates will need to be analyzed over longterm to evaluate outcomes. A meta-analysis of thoracoscopic neonatal CDH repairs illustrated that a thoracoscopic repair is associated with a 3-fold increased recurrence rate and longer operative times, although the mortality rate was similar in open and thoracoscopic repairs (Lansdale et al., 2010). Potentially, the thorocoscopic approach does not allow sufficient mobilization of the posterior leaflet of the diaphragm, committing more patients to prosthetic graft repairs overall.

5. Conclusion

In summary given the heterogeneity of disease severity, the complexity of CDH repairs has not been able to be prognostically separated into clear risk-stratified groups preoperatively to appropriately match for the therapies best suited to a category of risk. Now that the relationship of defect size to incidence of patch severity has been established, it is clear that many strategies are needed to best benefit those with the greatest defects and the worst CDH severity, both in the short term and long term. Composite bioprosthetic grafts and biologics have shown promise.

6. References

Baroncello JB, Czeczko NG, & Malafaia O (2008). The repair of abdominal defects in rabbits with Parietex and Surgisis meshes abdominal wall. *Arq Gastroenterol*, 45:323-9.

Bax NMA & Collins DL. (1984).The advantages of reconstruction of the dome of the diaphragm in congenital posterolateral diaphragmatic defects. *J Pediatr Surg*,19:484-7.

Brant- Zawadzki, PB, Fenton SJ., Nichol PF, Matlak ME, & Scaife ER. (2007). The split abdominal wall muscle flap repair for large congenital diaphragmatic hernias on extracorporeal membrane oxygenation. *J Pediatr Surg*, 42:1047-1051.

Bretelle F, Mazouni C, & D'Ercole C (2007) Fetal lung-head ratio measurement in the evaluation of congenital diaphragmatic hernia. *J Pediatr Surg*, 42:1312-1313.

Brindle ME, Brar M, & Skarsgard ED (2011)Patch repair is an independent predictor of morbidity and mortality in congenital diaphragmatic hernia. *Ped. Surg Int.*, 27:969-974.

Casaccia G, Crescenzi F & Dotta A(2006)Birthweight and McGoon Index predict mortality in newborn infants with congenital diaphragmatic hernia. *J Pediatr Surg*, 41:25-28.

Centers for Disease Control and Prevention. (2007) Hospital stays, hospital charges, and in-hospital deaths among infants with selected birth defects- United States, 2003. *MMWR Morb Mortal Wkly Rep*, 56:25-9.

Cho SD, Krishnaswami S & McKee JC (2009). Analysis of 29 consecutive thoracoscopic repairs of congenital diaphragmatic hernias in neonates compared to historical controls. *J Pediatr Surg*, 44:80-86.

Clark RH, Hardin WD Jr, & Hirschl RB (1998). Current surgical management of congenital diaphragmatic hernia: a report from the congenital diaphragmatic study group. *J Pediatr Surg*, 33:1004-1009.

Cohen D & Reid IS. (1981). Recurrent diaphragmatic hernia. *J Pediatr Surg* 1981;16:42-3.

Deprest JA, Flemmer AW & Gratacos E (2009).Antenatal prediction of lung volume and in utero treatment by fetal endoscopic tracheal occlusion in severe isolated CDH. *Sem Fetal Neonatal Med*,14:8-13.

Finer NN & Barrington KJ. (2001).Nitric Oxide for respiratory failure in infants born at or near term. *Cochrane Database Syst Rev*. CD000399.

Gonzalez R, Hill SJ& Wulkan ML. (2011). Absorbable versus Nonabsorbable mesh repair of congenital diaphragmatic hernia in a growing animal model. *J Laparoendosc Adv Surg Tech*, 21(5):449-454.

Graziano JN. (2005). Cardiac anomalies in patients with congenital diaphragmatic hernia and their prognosis: a report from the Congenital Diaphragmatic Hernia Study Group. *J Pediatr Surg*, 40:1045-1049.

Greig JD, Azmy AF. (1990) Thoracic cage deformity: A late complication following repair of an agenesis of diaphragm. *J Pediatr Surg*, 25:1234-1235.

Grethel EJ, Cortes RA, Wagner AJ & Clifton MS (2006). Prosthetic patches for congenital diaphragmatic hernia repair: Surgisis vs Gore-Tex. *J Pediatr Surg*, 41:29-33.

Harrison MR, Keller RL & Hawgood SB (2003). A randomized trial of fetal endoscopic tracheal occlusion for severe fetal congenital diaphragmatic hernia. *N Engl J Med*, 349:1916-1924.

Hajer GF, vd Staak FHJM & de Haan AFJ (1998). Recurrent congenital diaphragmatic hernia: which factors are involved. *Eur J Pediatr Surg*, 8:329-33

Hedrick HL, Danzer E & Merchant A (2007). Liver position and lung-to-head ratio for prediction of extracorporeal membrane oxygenation and survival in isolated left congenital diaphragmatic hernia. *Am J Obstet Gynecol*, 197(422):e421-424.

Hilfiker ML, Karamanoukian HL & Hudak M (1998). Congenital diaphragmatic hernia and chromosomal abnormalities: report of a lethal association. *Pediatr Surg Int*, 13:550-552.

Hirschl RB. (2004). Current Experience with liquid ventilation. *Paediatr Respir Rev*, 5 Suppl A:S339-S345.

Hunter L, Richens T, & Davis C (2009). Sildenafil use in congenital diaphragmatic hernia. *Arch Dis Child Fetal Neonatal Ed*, 94:F467

Jancelewicz T, Vu LT, Keller RL & Bratton B (2010). Long-term surgical outcomes in congenital diaphragmatic hernia: observations from a single institution. *J Pediatr Surg*, 45:155-160.

Keijzer R, Liu J & Deimling J (2000).Dual-hit hypothesis explains pulmonary hypoplasia in the nitrofen model of congenital diaphragmatic hernia. *Am J Pathol*, 156:1299-1306.

Khan AM & Lally KP. (2005).The role of extracorporeal membrane oxygenation in the management of infants with congenital diaphragmatic hernia. *Semin Perinatol*, 118-122.

Kim A, Bryner B & Akay B (2009). Thoroscopic repair of congenital diaphragmatic hernia in neonates: lessons learned. *J Laparoendosc Adv Surg Tech A*, 19:575-580.

Kitano Y, Okuyama H & Saito M (2011). Reevaluation of stomach position as a simple prognostic factor in fetal left congenital diaphragmatic hernia: a multicenter survey. *Ultrasound Obstet Gynecol*, 37(3): 277-282.

Kitano Y, Nakagawa S & Kuroda T (2005). Liver position in fetal congenital diaphragmatic hernia retains a prognostic value in the era of lung-protective strategy. *J Pediatr Surg*, 40:1827-1832.

Kunisaki SM, Barnewolt CE & Estroff JA (2008). Liver position is a prenatal predictive factor of prosthetic repair in congenital diaphragmatic hernia. *Fetal Diagn Ther*,23:258-262.

Lally KP, Lally PA & Lasky RE (2007). Defect size determines survival in infants with congenital diaphragmatic hernia. *Pediatrics*, 120:e651-657.

Lally KP, Lally PA & Langham MR (2004). Surfactant does not improve survival rate in preterm infants with congenital diaphragmatic hernia. *J Pediatr Surg*, 39 (6):829-33.

Langham MR, Kays DW & Beierle EA (2003). Twenty years of progress in congenital diaphragmatic hernia at the University of Florida. *Am Surg*, 69:45-52.

Lansdale N, Alam S, Losty PD & Jesudason EC. (2010). Neonatal Endosurgical Congenital Diaphragmatic Hernia Repair. *Ann of Surgery*, 252 (1):20-26.

Lantis II JC, Gallivan EK & Hekier R (2000). A comparison of collagen and PTFE patch repair in a rabbit model of congenital diaphragmatic hernia. *J Invest Surg*, 13:319-25.

Levison J, Halliday R & Holland AJA (2006). A population-based study of congenital diaphragmatic hernia outcome in New South Wales and the Australian Capital territory, Australia, 1992-2001. *J Ped Surg*, 41:1049-53.

Loff S, Wirth H & Jester I (2005). Implantation of a cone-shaped double-fixed patch increases abdominal space and prevents recurrence of large defects in congenital diaphragmatic hernia. *J Pediatr Surg*, 40:1701-1705.

Masumoto K, Nagata K & Souzaki R (2007). Effectiveness of diaphragmatic repair using an abdominal muscle flap in patients with recurrent congenital diaphragmatic hernia. *J Pediatr Surg*, 42;2007-11.

Miguet D, Claris O & Lapillonne A (1995). Preoperative stabilization using high-frequency oscillatory ventilation in the management of congenital diaphragmatic hernia. *Crit Care Med*, 22:887-92.

Mitchell IC, Garcia NM& Barber R (2008). Permacol: a potential biologic patch alternative in congenital diaphragmatic hernia repair. *J Pediatr Surg*, 43:2161-2164.

Mullassery D, Ba'ath ME & Jesudason EC (2010).Value of liver herniation in prediction of outcome in fetal congenital diaphragmatic hernia: a systematic review and meta-analysis. *Ultrasound Obst Gyn*, 35:609-614.

Moss RL, Chen CM & Harrison MR. (2001). Prosthetic patch durability in congenital diaphragmatic hernia: a long-term follow-up study. *J Ped. Surg*, 36:152-4.

Nasr A, Struijs M-C & P.L. Chiu. (2010). Outcomes after muscle flap vs prosthetic patch repair for large congenital diaphragmatic hernias. *J. Ped. Surg*, 45:151-154.

Nishie A, Tajima T & Asayama Y (2009). MR prediction of postnatal outcomes in left-sided congenital diaphragmatic hernia using right lung signal intensity: comparison with that using right lung volume. *J Magn Reson Imaging*, 30:112-120.

Okuyama H, Kubota A & Oue T(2002). Inhaled nitric oxide with early surgery improves the outcome of antenatally diagnosed congenital diaphragmatic hernia. *J Pediatr Surg*, 37:1188-1190.

Raval MV, Wang X, Reynolds M & Fischer AC. (2011) Costs of congenital diaphragmatic hernia repair in the United States-extracorporeal membrane oxygenation foots the bill. *J Pediatr Surg*. 46(4):617-24.

Richards SK, Lear PA & Huskisson L (2005). Porcine dermal collagen graft in pediatric transplantation. *Pediatr Transplant*, 9:627-9.

Riehle KJ, Magnunson DK & Waldhausen JH. (2007). Low recurrence rate after Gore-Tex/Marlex composite patch repair for posterolateral congenital diaphragmatic hernia. *J Pediatr Surg*, 42:1841-4.

Scaife ER, Johnson DG & Meyers RL (2003). The split abdominal wall muscle flap- A simple, mesh-free approach to repair large diaphragmatic hernia. *J Pediatr Surg*, 38:1748-51.

Shah S, Wishnew J, Barsness K & Gaines BA (2009). Minimally invasive congenital diaphragmatic hernia repair: a 7-year review of one institution's experience. *Surg Endosc*, 23:1265-1271.

Simpson JS & Gossage JD. (1971). Use of abdominal wall muscle flap in repair of large congenital diaphragmatic hernia. *J Pediatr Surg*, 6(1):42-44.

Singh SJ, Cummins GE & Cohen RC (1999). Adverse outcome of congenital diaphragmatic hernia is determined by diaphragmatic agenesis, not by antenatal diagnosis. *J Pediatr Surg*, 34:1740-1742.

Skargard ED, MacNab YC & Qiu Z (2005). SNAP-II predicts mortality among infants with congential diaphragmatic hernia. *J Perinatol*, 25:315-319.

Sola JE, Bronson SN & Cheung MC (2010). Survival disparities in newborns with congenital diaphragmatic hernia: a national perspective. *J Pediatr Surg*, 45:1336-1342.

Stege G, Fenton A & Jaffray B. (2004).Nihilism in the 1990s: the true mortality of congenital diaphragmatic hernia. *Pediatrics*, 112: 532-535.

St. Peter SD, Valusek PA & Tsao K (2007). Abdominal Complications related to type of repair for congenital diaphragmatic hernia. *J Surg Research*, 140:234-236.

Stringer MD, Goldstein RB & Filly RA (1995) Fetal diaphragmatic hernia without visceral herniation. *J Pediatr Surg*, 30(9):1264-6.

Sugiyama A, Fukumoto K & Fukuzawa H (2011). Free fascia lata repair for a second recurrent congenital diaphragmatic hernia. *J Pediatr Surg*, 46:1838-1841.

Sydorak RM, Hoffman H, Lee CD & Longaker M (2003). Reversed Latissimus Dorsi Muscle flap for repair of recurrent congenital diaphragmatic hernia. *J Pediatr Surg*, 38(3):296-300.

Tsao K, Lally PA & Lally KP.(2011). Minimally invasive repair of congenital diaphragmatic hernia. *J Pediatr Surg*, 46:1158-1164.

Valfre L, Braguglia A, Conforti A & Morini F (2011).Long term follow-up in high-risk congenital diaphragmatic hernia survivors: patching the diaphragm affects the outcome. *J Pediat Surg*, 46:52-56.

Vanamo K, Peltonen J & Rintala R (1996). Chest wall and spinal deformities in adults with congenital diaphragmatic defects. *J Pediatr Surg*, 31:851-4.

Witters I, Legius E & Moerman P(2001). Associated malformations and chromosomal anomalies in 42 cases of prenatally diagnosed diaphragmatic hernia. *Am J Med Genet*, 103:278-282.

Yang SH, Nobuhara KK & Keller RL (2007). Reliability of the lung-to-head ratio as a predictor of outcome in fetuses with isolated left congenital diaphragmatic hernia at gestation outside 24-26 weeks. *Am J Obst Gynecol*, 197:30.e1-37.

Yang EY, Allmendinger N, Johnson SM &Chen C (2005). Neonatal thoracoscopic repair of congenital diaphragmatic hernia: selection criteria for successful outcome. *J Ped Surg*, 40: 1369-1375.

Section 4

Outcomes for Children with Congenital Diaphragmatic Hernia

10

Congenital Diaphragmatic Hernia Survivors: Outcomes in Infancy, Childhood and Adolescence

Jennifer R. Benjamin[1] and C. Michael Cotten[2]
[1]*Yale University School of Medicine*
[2]*Duke University Medical Centre*
USA

1. Introduction

Congenital diaphragmatic hernia (CDH) remains highly challenging. CDH is complex and often results in multi-system morbidity among survivors. In the past decade, significant technologic and medical advancements have enhanced the care of critically ill infants, including those born with CDH. Such advancements have led to improved survival rates among CDH infants at certain high-volume centres, but this has occurred at the expense of increased short- and long-term morbidities for patients who previously would have died.

As collective knowledge has improved regarding the range of outcomes experienced by CDH survivors, the focus of much clinical research has shifted toward reducing survivor morbidity. Accordingly, many centres now offer multidisciplinary follow-up care for CDH survivors throughout infancy and early childhood in order to effectively diagnose and treat problems with the goal of maximizing the potential of the individual patient.

The aim of this chapter is to describe the short- and long-term medical and neurodevelopmental outcomes of CDH survivors in infancy, childhood, and adolescence. We will also outline an approach to follow-up care for these highly complex and intriguing patients.

2. Cardiopulmonary morbidity

Because the diaphragmatic defect allows abdominal organs to herniate into the chest cavity during the time of bronchial and pulmonary artery branching, lung growth and development are subsequently impaired. Long-term pulmonary morbidity is variable and depends on the degree of underlying pulmonary hypoplasia as well as the severity of iatrogenic injury the lungs incurred in the neonatal period. Treatment with extracorporeal membrane oxygenation (ECMO) and patch repair of the diaphragm are also associated with persistent cardiorespiratory complications (Jaillard et al., 2003; Muratore et al., 2001). Up to 50% of CDH survivors have long-lasting cardiopulmonary compromise, manifested as chronic lung disease, reactive airway disease, recurrent respiratory infections, and persistent pulmonary hypertension (Bagolan & Morini, 2007; Lally & Engle, 2008; Trachsel et al., 2005; Wischermann et al., 1995).

2.1 Chronic lung disease

Lung structure is fundamentally altered in CDH due to the decreased number of bronchi and alveoli in the ipsilateral and, to a lesser degree, contralateral lung. Although the number of alveoli may increase over time (Beals et al., 1992), the number of larger airways does not, because bronchial development is complete at around 16 weeks of gestation (Reid, 1984). Postnatally, exposure to supplemental oxygen and mechanical ventilation results in pulmonary edema and protein leak, causing surfactant denaturation and lung injury. The suboptimal nutrition often experienced by critically ill infants may further worsen the problem. Taken together, these factors lead to the development of chronic lung disease - a highly significant problem for between 40% and 60% of CDH survivors (D'Agostino et al., 1995; Kinsella et al., 1997; van den Hout et al., 2010).

D'Agostino et al documented a 62% incidence of chronic lung disease among ECMO-treated CDH survivors at hospital discharge (D'Agostino et al., 1995). Bernbaum et al found a similar incidence of 63% with bronchopulmonary dysplasia (BPD, a form of chronic lung disease) at discharge, with only a slight improvement to 50% at age one. Strikingly, four of seven CDH-ECMO patients in this report continued to need artificial ventilatory support at one year of age (Bernbaum et al., 1995). In a study of infants with pulmonary hypertension, Kinsella et al found CDH infants to have a 41% incidence of chronic lung disease; this incidence was significantly higher than the incidence of chronic lung disease due to meconium aspiration syndrome or respiratory distress syndrome, and suggests the possibility of decreased total lung volume combined with more severe underlying parenchymal lung disease in the CDH group (Kinsella et al., 1997). Van den Hout et al documented a 41% prevalence of BPD in a study of 2078 CDH patients based on data from the CDH Study Group. The authors identified early gestational age, presence of cardiac abnormality, prenatal diagnosis, right-sided defect, low 5-minute Apgar score, and intial treatment with high-frequency ventilation as factors predictive of BPD in CDH survivors. They suggest that in addition to injury from volutrauma, barotrauma, and atelectotrauma, the hypoplastic lungs in CDH may be more susceptible to oxygen toxicity than lungs of newborns with other respiratory disorders (van den Hout et al., 2010). Differences in definitions of respiratory morbidity among survivors makes comparison of heterogenous studies somewhat difficult, yet overall morbidity ranges between 30-50% in general (Table 1).

2.2 Reactive airway disease

Approximately 25% of CDH infants demonstrate evidence of obstructive airway disease (Jaillard et al., 2003), with up to 45% of survivors showing asthma-like symptoms during childhood and adolesence (Davis et al., 2004; Trachsel et al., 2005). A study by Crankson and colleagues found 45% of 31 CDH survivors had recurrent wheezing attacks and required bronchodilators and/or inhaled steroids (Crankson et al., 2005). In another report, bronchodilators were prescribed in 40% and inhaled steroids in 35% of CDH survivors during the first year of life (Muratore et al., 2001). Lung function abnormalities appear to improve over time as compensatory lung growth occurs, although these data are limited to a relatively small number of patients (Peetsold et al., 2007; Trachsel et al., 2005). According to some experts, although CDH survivors may exhibit mild to moderate abnormalities on pulmonary function testing in late childhood through adulthood, they appear *not* to have an important reduction of total lung capacity, and may be expected to achieve normal exercise function (Ijsselstijn et al., 1997; Marven et al., 1998; Peetsold et al., 2007).

Author, Year, Study Design	Definition	ECMO-treated	Age at Follow-up	Survival	Respiratory Morbidity
D'Agostino, et al. 1995 Single-center, retrospective	CLD: need for bronchodilators, diuretics, or supplemental oxygen for management of pulmonary symptoms	yes (all)	3, 6, and 12 months	80% at discharge (16 of 20)	62% at discharge (n=16) 30% at age 1 year (n=13)
Bernbaum, et al. 1995 Single-center, retrospective	BPD: (at discharge) greater than 30 days of supplemental oxygen and need for diuretics or bronchodilators for treatment of underlying CLD; (at follow-up) continued need for supplemental oxygen, diuretics, or bronchodilators	yes (all)	6 and 12 months	68% at discharge (19 of 28)	63% at discharge (n=19) 50% at age 1 year (n=14)
Kinsella, et al. 1997 Multicenter, randomized clinical trial	CLD: oxygen requirement at 28 days of age	yes (number not reported)	n/a	53% at discharge (18 of 34)	41% at day 28 (n=34)
van den Hout, et al. 2010 Multicenter, retrospective	BPD: oxygen requirement at 30 days of age	yes (29%)	n/a	76% at day 30 (1586 of 2078) 69% at discharge	41% at day 30 (n=1511)

Table 1. Definitions and outcomes for studies documenting chronic lung disease (CLD) and bronchopulmonary dysplasia (BPD) in CDH survivors

2.3 Oxygen dependency, respiratory infections, and tracheostomy

A 2001 report by Muratore et al found 16% of CDH survivors required supplemental oxygen at the time of hospital discharge; more recent studies show this number to be closer to 40% to 50% (Colby 2004; Cortes et al., 2005). Coughing and frequent respiratory infections occur in 25% to 50% of children, particularly in the first year of life (Falconer et al., 1990; Kamata et al., 2005). A significant percentage of CDH patients are discharged home on diuretic therapy for management of pulmonary edema (Muratore et al., 2001). Additionally, up to 4% of CDH infants ultimately require tracheostomy for respiratory failure in the setting of severe lung disease (Bagolan & Morini, 2007; Jaillard et al., 2003).

2.4 Pulmonary hypertension

Chronic pulmonary hypertension is one of the major complicating factors in CDH (Kinsella et al., 2005), and, according to one report, occurs in up to 21% of CDH infants (Kinsella et al., 2003). Recurrence of pulmonary hypertension beyond the neonatal period may lead to prolonged mechanical ventilation, a second ECMO run, or death (Dela Cruz et al., 1996; Lally & Breaux, 1995). In a small retrospective study of 8 infants with CDH, 100% were found to have evidence of pulmonary hypertension on echocardiography (Benjamin et al., 2010). Overall mortality attributable to pulmonary hypertension approaches 50% in the CDH population (Kinsella et al., 1997; The Neonatal Inhaled Nitric Oxide Study Group (NINOS), 1997).

In an attempt to correlate outcome with the severity of pulmonary hypertension among a cohort of CDH infants, Dillon et al investigated estimates of pulmonary artery pressures using serial echocardiography. Based on their findings, the authors propose that almost half of CDH patients will resolve their pulmonary hypertension within the first 21 days, and survival may be nearly 100% in this subpopulation. Conversely, a certain number of CDH infants will show persistent systemic or suprasystemic pressures despite all interventions (including ECMO), and survival among this group can be presumed zero. Finally, there exists a group with protracted pulmonary hypertension that is responsive to maximum medical management; survival rates for infants with this degree of pulmonary hypertension lie somewhere in between the two extremes (Dillon et al., 2004).

Schwartz et al investigated the outcome of 21 CDH-ECMO survivors at a mean age of 3.2 years and found 38% with pulmonary hypertension based on echocardiographic findings. Of those, 88% had some evidence of reactive airway disease and were on bronchodilators at the time of the study. There is, however, no mention of whether the patients were being treated with medication for pulmonary hypertension. The authors surmise that CDH infants may undergo a gradual increase in vascular smooth muscle proliferation leading to an increase in pulmonary arterial pressures over time. It remains unclear whether pulmonary vascular pressures eventually normalize as repair and growth progress (Schwartz et al., 1999).

Management strategies for CDH infants who do not require mechanical ventilation but have pulmonary hypertension include inhaled nitric oxide (iNO) via nasal cannula and oral sildenafil, a highly selective phosphodiesterase inhibitor type 5 (Keller et al., 2004; Kinsella et al., 2003). Sildenafil has been used to treat older children and adults with pulmonary hypertension (Wilkens et al., 2001) by limiting degradation of cyclic GMP and thereby enhancing endogenous nitric oxide activity (Tulloh, 2009). Results from a 2007 study indicate sildenafil may augment cardiac output in infants with CDH during the first two weeks of administration (Noori et al., 2007).

Though some reports document the presence of pulmonary hypertension in CDH beyond the neonatal period, little is known about the long-term structural pulmonary vascular abnormalities that remain, and how these structural abnormalities translate into clinical outcomes for older children and adults with chronic pulmonary hypertension following

CDH repair. More research is needed to assess the prevalence of persistent pulmonary hypertension, investigate the natural course of changing pulmonary pressures, determine the best methods for diagnosing pulmonary hypertension in CDH survivors, and determine the optimal dosing, timing, and indications for pharmacologic intervention.

3. Growth and nutritional morbidity

Numerous studies have documented the high incidence of gastrointestinal morbidity in CDH survivors (Fasching et al., 2000; Muratore et al., 2001; Van Meurs et al., 1993). Symptomatic gastroesophageal reflux (GER), feeding difficulties, and chronic growth failure necessitating supplemental enteral tube feedings are among the issues these infants and children face.

3.1 Gastroesophageal reflux

GER occurs in the vast majority of infants and children born with CDH, and is perhaps the most commonly encountered long-term problem among survivors. Several mechanisms have been proposed to explain the high incidence of GER in CDH, including fetal esophageal obstruction resulting in impaired esophageal motility, shortened esophageal length, disruption of the angle of His due to the abnormal location of the stomach *in utero,* and the complete or partial absence of the parahiatal diaphragm. The clinical presentation varies: some infants and children will experience recurrent vomiting, while in others GER may manifest as persistent bradycardic spells or aspiration pneumonia (Kieffer et al., 1995). Although many CDH survivors can be successfully managed with medical treatment, a significant number - up to 23% in one series - have severe GER requiring surgical intervention with fundoplication (Su et al., 2007). Factors associated with need for fundoplication are patch repair, ECMO treatment, and intrathoracic liver position (Diamond et al., 2007; Su et al., 2007).

Recently, Maier et al attempted to determine whether performing preventive fundoplication at the time of CDH repair would impact GER symptoms in infancy. The authors found a clinically (but not statistically) significant difference between the degree of GER in the first postnatal year among those infants who did (n = 36) and did not (n = 43) have preventive fundoplication performed at the time of hernia repair, but there was no difference by the second year of follow-up. These authors concluded that preventive anti-reflux surgery cannot be recommended as standard of care (Maier et al., 2011).

In contrast to the plethora of studies focusing on the gastrointestinal sequelae of CDH in infancy and childhood, there are relatively few studies describing outcomes among adult CDH survivors. Reports suggest a certain percentage of adult CDH survivors may have continued GER resulting in esophagitis and, in severe cases, Barrett's esophagus. Vanamo et al found 63% of adult survivors to have symptoms suggestive of GERD and 54% with evidence of esophagitis on endoscopy. Further, 2 of 11 patients with early postoperative GER developed esophageal stricture and underwent fundoplication (Vanamo et al., 1996). Steven et al described a case of esophageal adenocarcinoma in a 22 year-old CDH survivor; the malignancy was presumed to be related to long-standing GER associated with CDH (Steven et al., 2007). More studies are needed in adolescents and adults to determine whether the significant degree of GER experienced by CDH survivors in infancy and childhood remains a problem over time, and to what extent it impacts the health and wellbeing of adult survivors.

3.2 Feeding problems

Protracted hospitalization combined with symptoms of GER and delayed initiation of oral feedings contributes to the development of feeding difficulties in CDH infants. In one series, oral aversion was observed in 25% of infants with CDH and contributed largely to growth failure (Jaillard et al., 2003). Van Meurs et al found 22% of CDH-EMO survivors to have "extreme food refusal" in the first two years of life, 75% of whom required long-term supplemental nutrition. In general, one-third to one-half of CDH infants require supplementation with enteral tube feedings to support growth in the first year of life, either via nasogastric or gastrostomy tube feedings (Muratore et al., 2001; Van Meurs et al., 1993).

Symptoms of GER and resultant feeding problems may be more clinically apparent among CDH-ECMO survivors. In a study of 16 CDH-ECMO survivors, 81% were diagnosed with GER, and 69% were discharged requiring supplemental tube feedings (D'Agostino et al., 1995). Similarly, in Van Meurs' population of 18 CDH-ECMO survivors, at the time of hospital discharge, reflux precautions were in place for 22%, feedings were thickened with rice cereal for 22%, and 33% were being treated with metoclopramide (Van Meurs et al., 1993).

3.3 Failure to thrive

In conjunction with an increased metabolic demand due to pulmonary morbidity and underlying GER, feeding-related problems often result in failure to thrive. Muratore et al documented weight and height below the 25th percentile in more than 50% of CDH infants during the first year of life. In this study, ECMO treatment and need for oxygen at discharge were independent predictors of growth failure in the first postnatal year (Muratore et al., 2001). Others have similarly reported a relationship between ECMO and subsequent poor growth among CDH survivors; this finding is specific to the CDH-ECMO population, as non-CDH ECMO children were shown to have essentially normal growth at 12 and 24 months in Van Meurs' study (Nobuhara et al., 1996; Van Meurs et al., 1993). Further, Van Meurs et al found that parental discontinuation of supplemental tube feedings contributed to findings of severe malnourishment at one year follow-up (Van Meurs et al., 1993). A significant proportion of CDH survivors remain below the 5th percentile for weight in the first three years (Kamata et al., 2005; Lund et al., 1994). Catch-up growth can occur with aggressive management (Cortes et al., 2005), but poor growth remains a problem for a subset of patients.

4. Musculoskeletal morbidity

Chest wall and spinal deformities occur relatively commonly as a sequelae of CDH. One study of adult survivors found 48% with chest asymmetry, 27% with significant scoliosis, and 18% with pectus excavatum (Vanamo et al., 1996). The incidence increases with a larger diaphragmatic defect, presumably because repair of a large defect puts tension on the spine and interferes with normal development of the thorax. Other contributing factors include a smaller thoracic cavity on the affected side and increased work of breathing leading to development of a pectus abnormality via retraction of the cartilaginous anterior chest wall. For the most part, these deformities are mild and rarely require surgical intervention. However, the exact relationship between chest wall deformities and long-term pulmonary function remains unclear. Trachsel et al found a correlation between moderate to severe chest wall abnormalities and impaired pulmonary functioning in adulthood (Trachsel et al., 2005). Additionally, there is some evidence of abnormal lung function among patients with pectus excavatum (Koumbourlis & Stolar, 2004).

5. Surgical morbidity

The incidence of reherniation at the site of the diaphragmatic defect is directly related to the use of synthetic patch repair and ranges from 5% to 80% (Atkinson & Poon, 1992; Van Meurs et al., 1993). With the increasing popularity of minimally invasive surgical (MIS) techniques, studies have begun to investigate the short- and long-term outcomes following this approach. Using data from the CDH Study Group, Tsao et al looked at the in-hospital hernia recurrence rate following MIS and found a significantly higher proportion of recurrence in the MIS group compared with open repair; the authors estimated an almost 4-fold increased odds of recurrence with MIS repairs. In this study, infants who required a patch repair had a higher recurrence rate, and MIS repairs that used a patch had the highest recurrence rate of approximately 9% (Tsao et al., 2011). The overall benefit for MIS in CDH patients remains to be determined.

Timing of reherniation varies from months to years after the initial repair. Patients may present with gastrointestinal symptoms (feeding difficulties, vomiting), respiratory symptoms (coughing, wheezing), or they may be asymptomatic. Thus, regularly scheduled surveillance chest radiographs are advised (Lally & Engle, 2008; Moss et al., 2001).

Almost invariably, infants with CDH have intestinal non-rotation or malrotation. Consequently, some are at risk for developing intestinal obstruction due to midgut volvulus if a Ladd's procedure was not performed at the time of diaphragmatic repair. Postoperative intra-abdominal adhesions may also lead to intestinal obstruction - a life-threatening complication if not recognized and treated in a timely manner.

6. Neurodevelopmental morbidity

The underlying mechanisms of brain injury in CDH remain incompletely defined. Chronic lung disease, postnatal growth failure, and prolonged hospitalization are factors known to adversely affect neurodevelopment. In addition, most infants with CDH are exposed to perinatal and postnatal hypoxia, hypotension, hypercapnia, inflammation, and acidosis - all of which interfere with central nervous system development. Poor neurodevelopmental outcome in infants with CDH is likely the result of a combination of multiple interrelated factors. All CDH survivors should be considered at risk for cognitive delay and followed regularly in a multidisciplinary clinic.

6.1 Neurodevelopmental outcomes among non-ECMO-treated CDH survivors

In spite of heightened awareness about the potential for long-lasting adverse neurodevelopmental outcome in CDH survivors, most studies have focused on the 18- to 36-month follow up period, with a considerable paucity of information detailing longer-term outcomes. Similarly, few studies describe the neurodevelopmental outcome of CDH survivors *not* treated with ECMO. Only recently have investigators begun to look at the developmental and psychological outcomes of survivors into late childhood and adolescence.

One such series looking at CDH survivors between 8 and 12 years of age found only 54% to be functioning cognitively at expected school level. In addition, there was a higher prevalence of emotional and behavioural problems among survivors in comparison to the general population (Bouman et al., 2000). In a study of adolescent CDH survivors, Jakobson and colleagues studied the visual and fine motor outcomes of CDH survivors between ages 10 through 16 and found 13% had severe cognitive impairment, with the majority of the remaining showing poorer oral motor control and visual-motor integration skills as compared to peers (Jakobson et al., 2009). Notably, none of the survivors in these two studies were treated with ECMO as infants.

6.2 Neurodevelopmental outcomes among CDH-ECMO survivors

The relationship between CDH infants treated with ECMO and adverse neurocognitive outcome remains controversial. Some experts conclude that although ECMO can support the most critically ill infants, its use in the CDH population is associated with significant mortality and long-term morbidity (Bernbaum et al., 2005; Davis et al., 2004). On the contrary, others question whether adverse outcomes in this population may be due to the underlying disease process or an intrinsic neurologic abnormality rather than ECMO per se (D'Agostino et al., 1995; Jaillard et al., 2003; Lally & Engle, 2008).

The physiologic basis for ECMO treatment leading to cognitive delay rests on several factors. First, infants who require ECMO to survive represent the sickest subset of patients in the newborn intensive care unit (NICU). They are at significant risk for hypoxia and hypoperfusion before and during ECMO treatment (Bagolan & Morini, 2007) and, therefore, are very likely subject to hypoxic-ischemic brain injury. Furthermore, ECMO support requires systemic anticoagulation (in all) and ligation of the carotid artery (in venoarterial). The increase in neurologic complications in infants treated with venoarterial ECMO (seizures, cerebral infarction) may be attributable to decreased cerebral blood flow resulting from ligation of the right internal carotid artery (Dimmitt et al., 2001). One report suggests that venovenous ECMO may be sufficient to support CDH patients, and when compared with venoarterial ECMO, is associated with decreased risk of neurologic impairment (Guner et al., 2009).

A study by Van Meurs et al focusing on the outcome of 18 CDH-ECMO survivors between ages one and four years, 15 of whom underwent developmental testing, found 46% of the group to be normal, 20% with suspected developmental delays, and 13% with definitely abnormal developmental outcome (Van Meurs et al., 1993). In a report by Nobuhara and colleagues, 37% of 78 CDH survivors had developmental delay at follow-up; notably, 72% of the survivors with mild to moderate delays were treated with ECMO as neonates (Nobuhara et al., 1996). Similarly, McGahren et al described a statistically significant difference in neurologic abnormalities between CDH survivors who were and were not treated with ECMO: 67% of 12 CDH-ECMO infants had evidence of significant neurologic deficit at follow-up compared with 24% of 21 non-ECMO-treated CDH survivors (McGahren et al., 1997).

A 2004 study of CDH-ECMO survivors found 19% to have severe neurodevelopmental problems, defined as speech, language, or motor delay, at a median age of 5 years. In this report, only 25% of 27 CDH children were free of significant neurodevelopmental deficit at follow-up (Davis et al., 2004). Similarly, among 149 5 year-old ECMO survivors, Nijhuis-van der Sanden et al found the 36 with CDH to have the worst outcomes: nearly 42% died, 72% had growth problems, and almost 16% had severe disabilities with only 37% functioning normally (Nijhuis-van der Sanden et al., 2009). A recent study of 41 infants prospectively enrolled in an interdisciplinary follow-up program found 46% of CDH-ECMO survivors had deficits in developmental outcome at 24 months as well as an increased risk for psychomotor dysfunction and motor delays. Autism was diagnosed in 7% of this cohort (Danzer et al., 2010).

Several studies document the relationship between ECMO and hypotonia in infancy and early childhood. A report by D'Agostino and colleagues followed 13 CDH-ECMO survivors into early childhood and found a significant number to have problems with hypotonia, which subsequently had a large impact on motor skill acquisition. Fifty-four percent had normal cognitive and motor outcomes at 12 months while 23% had delays in both areas (D'Agostino et al., 1995). In Nobuhara's study, decreased lower extremity tone was the most common finding among CDH survivors with developmental delay (Nobuhara et al., 1996). Bernbaum et al studied a cohort of ECMO survivors and found the CDH-ECMO population to have significantly lower motor and slightly lower cognitive scores at one year of age compared with groups treated with ECMO for other reasons. In this study, 75% percent of CDH-ECMO infants with hypotonia at discharge continued to be hypotonic at age one, which affected the attainment of gross motor skills (Bernbaum et al., 1995).

In a study by Tracy et al looking at the relationship between neuroimaging abnormalities and neurodevelopmental outcomes in a cohort of 45 CDH survivors, the authors found hypotonia to be the most frequently noted neurologic finding on physical examination. Hypotonia was present in 37% of survivors at age one and 71% of survivors at age three years. Motor problems seemed to be associated with hypotonia, as motor problems were diagnosed in 46% and 71% of the cohort at ages one and three, respectively. Additionally, motor problems at one year of age were correlated with abnormal findings on postnatal neuroimaging, continued respiratory compromise at age one, and a history of prolonged mechanical ventilation (Tracy et al., 2010).

6.3 School-age follow-up of CDH survivors

In a study looking at predictors of neurocognitive delay among a cohort of 16 school-age CDH survivors, 44% of the study population had evidence of persistent neurocognitive delay between ages 4 and 7 years. In this study, eight subjects underwent developmental testing at both 2 year and school age follow-up, and 50% had evidence of both early impairment and continued delay at school age. The remaining four subjects who scored within the average range on neurodevelopmental testing at 2 years remained with average scores at early school age. We found patch repair, ECMO treatment, days on ECMO, days of mechanical ventilation, and post-operative use of iNO to be associated with neurocognitive delay at early school age (Benjamin et al., 2010).

6.4 Neuroimaging in CDH

As brain imaging techniques have become more widely available, researchers have begun to study the effects of CDH on the developing central nervous system. A study looking at eight CDH survivors - none treated with ECMO - found all to have abnormalities on brain MRI, including ventricular dilatation, abnormal myelination of the posterior limb of the internal capsule, and abnormal signal in the white matter and basal ganglia (Hunt et al., 2004). Tracy et al showed that by age three years, 88% of CDH survivors who underwent brain MRI studies had abnormal imaging findings, including extra axial fluid and periventricular leukomalacia. Additionally, abnormalities were present in 79% of those who underwent head computed tomography (CT) as a mode of neuroimaging (Tracy et al., 2010). Similarly, among a cohort of CDH-ECMO infants, 35% had central nervous system abnormalities on CT scan or at autopsy, including ventricular dilatation, intracranial hemorrhage, and cerebral atrophy. At two-year follow-up, the survivors were noted to have low-average scores on cognitive and motor testing (Ahmed et al., 1999).

6.5 Sensorineural hearing loss

Infants with CDH are known to be at high risk for sensorineural hearing loss (SNHL), though the precise etiology remains incompletely understood. In one of the earliest reports looking at infants with SNHL, Nield et al linked acidosis and severe hypoxia with the disease (Nield et al., 1986). In a study of infants with persistent pulmonary hypertension, alkalosis and prolonged duration of mechanical ventilation were found to be contributing factors (Hendricks-Munoz & Walton, 1988). In addition, high-frequency ventilation has been associated with SNHL (Lasky et al., 1998).

The incidence of SNHL has been reported in up to 60% of CDH survivors in one report (Morini et al., 2008), and up to 100% in another (Robertson et al., 2002). It must be underscored that up to 50% infants labeled as having normal hearing may develop hearing loss later in infancy (Fligor et al., 2005; Robertson et al., 2002). This type of hearing loss is progressive, and therefore, for all infants with CDH, repeated hearing screening at 6-month intervals throughout infancy and early childhood is indicated to prevent significant speech and language delay.

Among CDH infants, several reports link ECMO as a causative factor for the development of SNHL (Fligor et al., 2005; Nobuhara et al., 1996). A study by Rasheed et al found 100% of infants who were stabilized on ECMO pre-repair wore hearing aids compared with 22% who were treated with ECMO post-operatively. The authors suggest the difference may have been due to prolonged ECMO duration, more significant degrees of alkalosis and hyperventilation, and longer exposure to loop diuretics in the pre-repair group (Rasheed et al., 2001). Along with hypoxia and ECMO treatment, ototoxic medications commonly used in the NICU such as aminoglycoside antibiotics, loop diuretics, and neuromuscular blocking agents contribute to the high incidence of SHNL in this population (Masumoto et al., 2007).

Overall, long-term neurodevelopmental morbidity among CDH survivors is highest among those who require patch repair and those treated with ECMO. Whether this is reflective of more severe primary disease or due to the greater number of associated complications in those two groups remains a subject of debate. In fact, multiple factors likely contribute to long-term morbidity, including perinatal, perioperative, and other postnatal events. The need for further studies to determine the role of ECMO in the CDH population is paramount in order to ensure the best outcomes for the majority of patients.

7. Standardized treatment protocols for management of CDH

Recently, studies have shown that standardized treatment protocols improve outcomes among critically ill patients by allowing more consistent care and reducing variability in decision-making practices (Delaney et al., 2008; Holcomb et al., 2001; Morris, 2003).

Although a universal approach to management of the CDH infant does not yet exist, several authors have documented their successes after adopting centre-specific CDH management protocols. In one such report, the authors demonstrate that the institution of a treatment protocol is independently associated with decreased mortality risk among infants with CDH; in their study survival rates increased significantly from 67% to 88% following implementation of the protocol (van den Hout et al., 2011). Tracy et al noted similar results after the development and execution of an evidence-based care protocol for CDH infants, with survival to discharge improving from 55% to 85% despite comparable expected survival rates between the pre-protocol and protocol groups (Tracy et al., 2010).

With the aim of providing European neonatologists and pediatric intensive care physicians with a protocolized approach to the infant with CDH, the European task force for CDH (CDH EURO Consortium) recently drafted and published a consensus statement describing a standardized management protocol for CDH (Reiss et al., 2010). One may hope that a similar consensus statement will soon be realized in the United States and worldwide to allow more streamlined and evidence-based care for these highly complex patients.

Given the small numbers of CDH cases occurring at individual centres, cooperation and collaboration between centres and internationally is essential to develop such protocols, and to enhance further research in this field via randomized controlled trials and investigation into long-term outcomes among survivors (van den Hout et al., 2011; Wright et al., 2011).

8. Comprehensive follow-up for CDH survivors

Prior to leaving the hospital, standard discharge practices should be applied to infants with CDH, including measurement of weight, length, and head circumference, physical and neurologic examinations, and newborn hearing screening. Pre-discharge chest radiography may be helpful for comparision over time and to monitor for asymptomatic reherniation at the repair site. An echocardiogram should be considered to evaluate for residual pulmonary hypertension and/or persistent elevations in right-sided heart pressures. Neuroimaging (brain MRI or head CT) may be considered for infants with abnormalities on ultrasound or neurologic examination, and for all ECMO survivors. For the CDH infant with symptomatic GER, imaging studies may be useful in delineating the severity of the problem to aid in deciding whether surgical intervention is warranted. All routine newborn immunizations, including pneumococal and influenza vaccines, should be administered according to recommeded guidelines. In addition, CDH survivors with chronic lung disease are suggested to receive palivizumab (Synagis) for prophylaxis against respiratory syncytial virus (American Academy of Pediatrics, 2009).

Infants with CDH require long-term periodic follow-up evaluation to identify and effectively treat potential challenges; the goal is early and appropriate intervention to prevent additional disability and maximize developmental and cognitive outcomes. Ideally, this would be provided by a multidisciplinary team in a structured neonatal follow-up program in order to enhance communication and collaboration among providers while allowing the most comprehensive care possible. If such a program is not available, follow-up appointments should be arranged with the infant's primary care provider and with pediatric surgery at minimum. Follow-up with other specialists such as pediatric cardiology, pediatric neurology, and developmental-behavioral pediatrics should be arranged on an as-needed basis depending on the infant's degree of illness.

An article from the Section on Surgery and the Committee on Fetus and Newborn of the American Academy of Pediatrics advises that children with CDH be followed into adolescence to be sure that they are healthy and developing to the best of their potential. The Academy recommends specific medical tests as standard of care for CDH survivors, and the article includes a suggested schedule of follow-up, including annual neurodevelopmental screening and evaluation through school age (Table 2, Lally & Engle, 2008).

	Before Discharge	1-3 mo After Birth	4-6 mo After Birth	9-12 mo After Birth	15-18 mo After Birth	Annual Through 16 y
Weight, length, occipital-frontal circumference	X	X	X	X	X	X
Chest radiograph	X	If patched	If patched	If patched	If patched	If patched
Pulmonary function testing			If indicated		If indicated	If indicated
Childhood immunizations	As indicated throughout childhood	X	X	X	X	X
RSV prophylaxis	RSV season during first 2 years after birth (if evidence of chronic lung disease)	X	X	X	X	X
Echocardiogram and cardiology follow-up	X	If previously abnormal or on supple-mental oxygen	If previously abnormal or on supple-mental oxygen	If previously abnormal or on supple-mental oxygen	If previously abnormal or on supple-mental oxygen	If previously abnormal or on supple-mental oxygen
Head computed tomography or MRI	If (1) abnormal finding on head ultrasound; (2) seizures /abnormal neurologic findings; or (3) ECMO or patch repair	As indicated	As indicated	As indicated	As indicated	As indicated

	Before Discharge	1-3 mo After Birth	4-6 mo After Birth	9-12 mo After Birth	15-18 mo After Birth	Annual Through 16 y
Hearing evaluation	Auditory brainstem evoked response or otoacoustic emissions screen	X	X	X	X	Every 6 mo to age 3 y, then annually to age 5 y
Developmental screening evaluation	X	X	X	X		Annually to age 5 y
Neurodevelop-mental evaluation	X			X		Annually to age 5 y
Assessment for oral feeding problems	X	X	If oral feeding problems	If oral feeding problems	If oral feeding problems	If oral feeding problems
Upper gastrointestinal study, pH probe, and/or gastric scintiscan	Consider for all patients	If symptoms	If symptoms	Consider for all patients	If symptoms	If symptoms
Esophagoscopy		If symptoms	If symptoms	If symptoms or if abnormal gastro-intestinal evaluations	If symptoms	If symptoms
Scoliosis and chest wall deformity screening (physical examination, chest radiograph, and/or computed tomography of the chest)				X		X

Abbreviations: RSV, respiratory syncytial virus; CT, computed tomography; MRI, magnetic resonance imaging; ECMO, extracorporeal membrane oxygenation; GI, gastrointestinal. The neurosensory tests performed and frequency of surveillance may differ among infants because of variability in neurologic, developmental, and physiologic impairments. Follow-up should be tailored to each infant.
Reproduced with permission from *Pediatrics*, Vol. 121, Pages 627-632, © 2008 by the American Academy of Pediatrics.

Table 2. Recommended Schedule of Follow-up for Infants with CDH

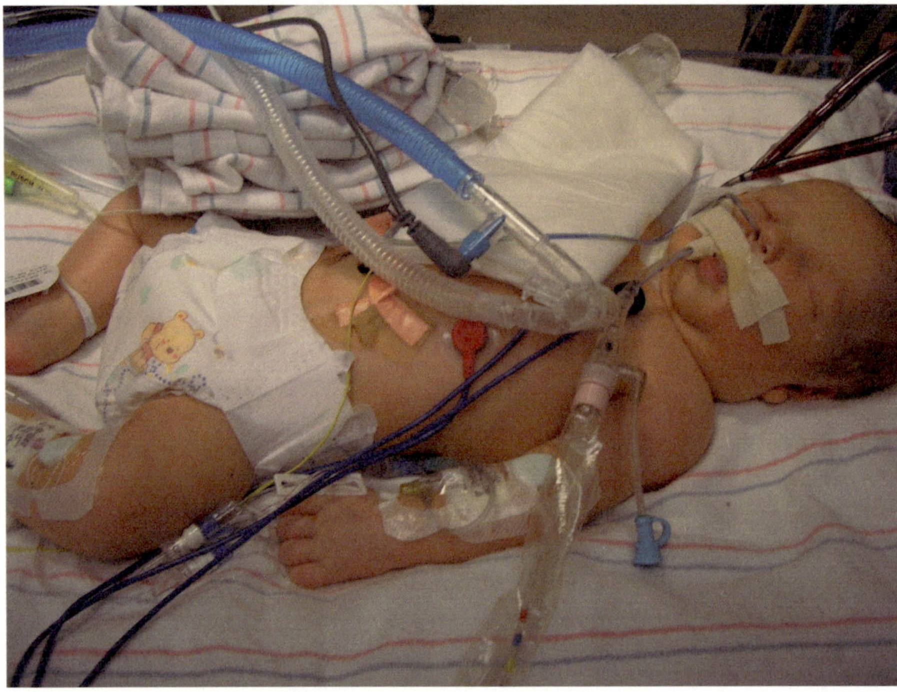

Fig. 1. JCM, 9 day old term infant with CDH, on VA ECMO for 18 days, hospitalized for 115 days.

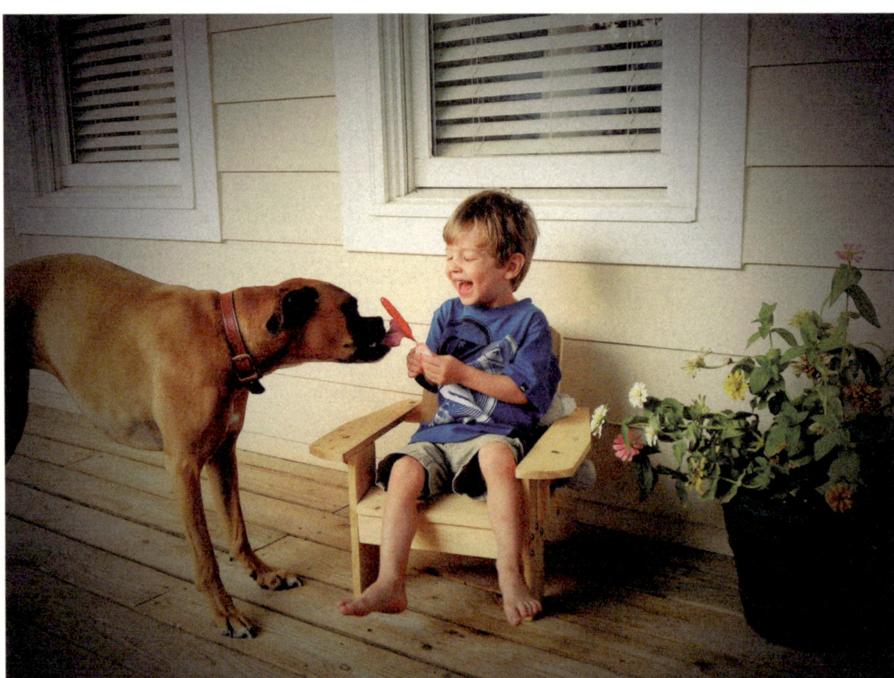

Fig. 2. JCM, CDH-ECMO survivor, age 2 ½, sharing a treat with his pal Lucy.

9. Conclusion

CDH occurs because of a deceivingly simple anatomic defect; however, its effects often lead to severe consequences and lasting implications for affected infants and their families. Advancements in pediatric surgery and neonatal intensive care have led to improved overall survival in high-volume centres, but at the expense of increased long-term morbidity in survivors. Research is ongoing, particularly in search of an *in utero* cure for CDH, but also regarding the long-term outcomes of survivors as they progress through infancy and childhood to become adolescents and adults with CDH.

CDH survivors provide a unique sense of satisfaction and joy to those who care for them; despite the difficulties, the potential for lasting health and well-being is great. These patients demand and deserve a multidisciplinary approach, both in the inpatient arena and follow-up setting, with experts in neonatology, surgery, pulmonology, cardiology, and neurodevelopment working together to optimize outcomes and determine how to achieve the highest survival rates while allowing the best possible long-term outcomes for those who survive.

10. References

Ahmad, A., Gangitano, E., Odell, R. M., Doran, R., & Durand, M. (1999). Survival, intracranial lesions, and neurodevelopmental outcome in infants with congenital diaphragmatic hernia treated with extracorporeal membrane oxygenation. *J Perinatol,* 19(6 Pt 1), 436-440.

American Academy of Pediatrics, Committee on Infectious Diseases. (2009). Modified Recommendations for Use of Palivizumab for Prevention of Respiratory Syncytial Virus Infections. *Pediatrics,* 124(6), 1694-1701.

Atkinson, J. B., & Poon, M. W. (1992). ECMO and the management of congenital diaphragmatic hernia with large diaphragmatic defects requiring a prosthetic patch. *Journal of Pediatric Surgery,* 27(6), 754-756.

Bagolan, P., & Morini, F. (2007). Long-term follow up of infants with congenital diaphragmatic hernia. *Semin Pediatr Surg,* 16(2), 134-144.

Beals, D. A., Schloo, B. L., Vacanti, J. P., Reid, L. M., & Wilson, J. M. (1992). Pulmonary growth and remodeling in infants with high-risk congenital diaphragmatic hernia. *Journal of Pediatric Surgery,* 27(8), 997-1002.

Benjamin, J. R., Jean-Baptiste, N., Goldberg, R. N., Smith, P. B., Cotten, C. M. (2010). Use of oral sildenafil for treatment of pulmonary hypertension in infants with congenital diaphragmatic hernia [abstr]. Presented at the Society for Pediatric Research, Vancouver, Canada.

Benjamin, J. R., Gustafson K. E., Smith, P. B., Ellingsen, K. M., Tompkins, K. B., Goldberg, R. N., Cotten, C. M., & Goldstein, R. F. (2010). Early school age follow-up of congenital diaphragmatic hernia survivors [abstr]. Presented at the Southeastern Regional Conference on Perinatal Research, Key Largo, FL.

Bernbaum, J., Schwartz, I. P., Gerdes, M., D'Agostino, J. A., Coburn, C. E., & Polin, R. A. (1995). Survivors of extracorporeal membrane oxygenation at 1 year of age: the relationship of primary diagnosis with health and neurodevelopmental sequelae. *Pediatrics,* 96(5 Pt 1), 907-913.

Bouman, N. H., Koot, H. M., Tibboel, D., & Hazebroek, F. W. (2000). Children with congenital diaphragmatic hernia are at risk for lower levels of cognitive functioning and increased emotional and behavioral problems. *Eur J Pediatr Surg,* 10(1), 3-7.

Colby, C. E. (2004). Surfactant replacement therapy on ECMO does not improve outcome in neonates with congenital diaphragmatic hernia. *Journal of Pediatric Surgery,* 39(11), 1632-1637.

Cortes, R. A., Keller, R. L., Townsend, T., Harrison, M. R., Farmer, D. L., Lee, H., et al. (2005). Survival of severe congenital diaphragmatic hernia has morbid consequences. *J Pediatr Surg,* 40(1), 36-45.

Crankson, S. J., Al Jadaan, S. A., Namshan, M. A., Al-Rabeeah, A. A., & Oda, O. (2006). The immediate and long-term outcomes of newborns with congenital diaphragmatic hernia. *Pediatr Surg Int,* 22(4), 335-340.

D'Agostino, J. A., Bernbaum, J. C., Gerdes, M., Schwartz, I. P., Coburn, C. E., Hirschl, R. B., et al. (1995). Outcome for infants with congenital diaphragmatic hernia requiring extracorporeal membrane oxygenation: The first year. *Journal of Pediatric Surgery,* 30(1), 10-15.

Danzer, E., Gerdes, M., Bernbaum, J., D'Agostino, J., Bebbington, M. W., Siegle, J., et al. (2010). Neurodevelopmental outcome of infants with congenital diaphragmatic hernia prospectively enrolled in an interdisciplinary follow-up program. *Journal of Pediatric Surgery,* 45(9), 1759-1766.

Davis, P. J., Firmin, R. K., Manktelow, B., Goldman, A. P., Davis, C. F., Smith, J. H., et al. (2004). Long-term outcome following extracorporeal membrane oxygenation for congenital diaphragmatic hernia: the UK experience. *The Journal of Pediatrics,* 144(3), 309-315.

Dela Cruz, T. V., Stewart, D. L., Robinson, T. W., & Bond, S. J. (1996). The use of a second course of extracorporeal membrane oxygenation in neonatal patients. *ASAIO Journal,* 42(3), 230-232.

Delaney, A., Angus, D. C., Bellomo, R., Cameron, P., Cooper, D. J., Finfer, S., et al. (2008). Bench-to-bedside review: the evaluation of complex interventions in critical care. *Crit Care,* 12(2), 210.

Diamond, I. R., Mah, K., Kim, P. C. W., Bohn, D., Gerstle, J. T., & Wales, P. W. (2007). Predicting the need for fundoplication at the time of congenital diaphragmatic hernia repair. *Journal of Pediatric Surgery,* 42(6), 1066-1070.

Dillon, P. W., Cilley, R. E., Mauger, D., Zachary, C., & Meier, A. (2004). The relationship of pulmonary artery pressure and survival in congenital diaphragmatic hernia. *Journal of Pediatric Surgery,* 39(3), 307-312.

Dimmitt, R. A., Moss, R. L., Rhine, W. D., Benitz, W. E., Henry, M. C. W., & VanMeurs, K. P. (2001). Venoarterial versus venovenous extracorporeal membrane oxygenation in congenital diaphragmatic hernia: The extracorporeal life support organization registry, 1990-1999. *Journal of Pediatric Surgery,* 36(8), 1199-1204.

Falconer, A. R., Brown, R. A., Helms, P., Gordon, I., & Baron, J. A. (1990). Pulmonary sequelae in survivors of congenital diaphragmatic hernia. *Thorax,* 45(2), 126-129.

Fasching, G., Huber, A., Uray, E., Sorantin, E., Lindbichler, F., & Mayr, J. (2000). Gastroesophageal reflux and diaphragmatic motility after repair of congenital diaphragmatic hernia. *European Journal of Pediatric Surgery,* 10(6), 360-364.

Guner, Y. S., Khemani, R. G., Qureshi, F. G., Wee, C. P., Austin, M. T., Dorey, F., et al. (2009). Outcome analysis of neonates with congenital diaphragmatic hernia treated with venovenous vs venoarterial extracorporeal membrane oxygenation. *J Pediatr Surg,* 44(9), 1691-1701.

Hendricks-Munoz, K. D., & Walton, J. P. (1988). Hearing loss in infants with persistent fetal circulation. *Pediatrics,* 81(5), 650-656.

Holcomb, B. W., Wheeler, A. P., & Ely, E. W. (2001). New ways to reduce unnecessary variation and improve outcomes in the intensive care unit. *Curr Opin Crit Care,* 7(4), 304-311.

Hunt, R. W., Kean, M. J., Stewart, M. J., & Inder, T. E. (2004). Patterns of cerebral injury in a series of infants with congenital diaphragmatic hernia utilizing magnetic resonance imaging. *Journal of Pediatric Surgery,* 39(1), 31-36.

Ijsselstijn, H., Tibboel, D., Hop, W. J., Molenaar, J. C., & de Jongste, J. C. (1997). Long-term pulmonary sequelae in children with congenital diaphragmatic hernia. *American Journal of Respiratory and Critical Care Medicine,* 155(1), 174-180.

Jakobson, L. S., Frisk, V., Trachsel, D., & O'Brien, K. (2009). Visual and fine-motor outcomes in adolescent survivors of high-risk congenital diaphragmatic hernia who did not receive extracorporeal membrane oxygenation. *Journal of Perinatology,* 29(9), 630-636.

Jaillard, S. M., Pierrat, V., Dubois, A., Truffert, P., Lequien, P., Wurtz, A. J., et al. (2003). Outcome at 2 years of infants with congenital diaphragmatic hernia: a population-based study. *Ann Thorac Surg,* 75(1), 250-256.

Kamata, S., Usui, N., Kamiyama, M., Tazuke, Y., Nose, K., Sawai, T., et al. (2005). Long-term follow-up of patients with high-risk congenital diaphragmatic hernia. *J Pediatr Surg,* 40(12), 1833-1838.

Keller, R. L., Hamrick, S. E. G., Kitterman, J. A., Fineman, J. R., & Hawgood, S. (2004). Treatment of rebound and chronic pulmonary hypertension with oral sildenafil in an infant with congenital diaphragmatic hernia. *Pediatric Critical Care Medicine,* 5(2), 184-187.

Kinsella, J. P., Parker, T. A., Ivy, D. D., & Abman, S. H. (2003). Noninvasive delivery of inhaled nitric oxide therapy for late pulmonary hypertension in newborn infants with congential diaphragmatic hernia. *The Journal of Pediatrics,* 142(4), 397-401.

Kinsella, J. P., Truog, W. E., Walsh, W. F., Goldberg, R. N., Bancalari, E., Mayock, D. E., et al. (1997). Randomized, multicenter trial of inhaled nitric oxide and high-frequency oscillatory ventilation in severe, persistent pulmonary hypertension of the newborn. *Journal of Pediatrics,* 131(1 Pt 1), 55-62.

Kinsella, J. P., Ivy, D. D., & Abman, S. H. (2005). Pulmonary Vasodilator Therapy in Congenital Diaphragmatic Hernia: Acute, Late, and Chronic Pulmonary Hypertension. *Seminars in Perinatology,* 29(2), 123-128.

Koumbourlis, A. C., & Stolar, C. J. (2004). Lung growth and function in children and adolescents with idiopathic pectus excavatum. *Pediatric Pulmonology,* 38(4), 339-343.

Lally, K. P., & Breaux, C. W., Jr. (1995). A second course of extracorporeal membrane oxygenation in the neonate--is there a benefit? *Surgery,* 117(2), 175-178.

Lally, K. P., & Engle, W. (2008). Postdischarge follow-up of infants with congenital diaphragmatic hernia. *Pediatrics,* 121(3), 627-632.

Lasky, R. E., Wiorek, L., & Becker, T. R. (1998). Hearing loss in survivors of neonatal extracorporeal membrane oxygenation (ECMO) therapy and high-frequency oscillatory (HFO) therapy. *Journal of the American Academy of Audiology*, 9(1), 47-58.

Lund, D. P., Mitchell, J., Kharasch, V., Quigley, S., Kuehn, M., & Wilson, J. M. (1994). Congenital diaphragmatic hernia: the hidden morbidity. *J Pediatr Surg*, 29(2), 258-262; discussion 262-254.

Maier, S., Zahn, K., Wessel, L. M., Schaible, T., Brade, J., & Reinshagen, K. (2011). Preventive antireflux surgery in neonates with congenital diaphragmatic hernia: a single-blinded prospective study. *Journal of Pediatric Surgery*, 46(8), 1510-1515.

Marven, S. S., Smith, C. M., Claxton, D., Chapman, J., Davies, H. A., Primhak, R. A., et al. (1998). Pulmonary function, exercise performance, and growth in survivors of congenital diaphragmatic hernia. *Archives of Disease in Childhood*, 78(2), 137-142.

Masumoto, K., Nagata, K., Uesugi, T., Yamada, T., & Taguchi, T. (2007). Risk factors for sensorineural hearing loss in survivors with severe congenital diaphragmatic hernia. *European Journal of Pediatrics*, 166(6), 607-612.

McGahren, E. D., Mallik, K., & Rodgers, B. M. (1997). Neurological outcome is diminished in survivors of congenital diaphragmatic hernia requiring extracorporeal membrane oxygenation. *J Pediatr Surg*, 32(8), 1216-1220.

Morini, F., Capolupo, I., Masi, R., Ronchetti, M. P., Locatelli, M., Corchia, C., et al. (2008). Hearing impairment in congenital diaphragmatic hernia: the inaudible and noiseless foot of time. *J Pediatr Surg*, 43(2), 380-384.

Morris, A. H. (2003). Treatment algorithms and protocolized care. *Curr Opin Crit Care*, 9(3), 236-240.

Moss, L. R., Chen, C. M., & Harrison, M. R. (2001). Prosthetic patch durability in congenital diaphragmatic hernia: A long-term follow-up study. *Journal of Pediatric Surgery*, 36(1), 152-154.

Muratore, C. S., Utter, S., Jaksic, T., Lund, D. P., & Wilson, J. M. (2001). Nutritional morbidity in survivors of congenital diaphragmatic hernia. *J Pediatr Surg*, 36(8), 1171-1176.

Muratore, C. S., Kharasch, V., Lund, D. P., Sheils, C., Friedman, S., Brown, C., et al. (2001). Pulmonary morbidity in 100 survivors of congenital diaphragmatic hernia monitored in a multidisciplinary clinic. *J Pediatr Surg*, 36(1), 133-140.

The Neonatal Inhaled Nitric Oxide Study Group (NINOS). (1997). Inhaled Nitric Oxide and Hypoxic Respiratory Failure in Infants With Congenital Diaphragmatic Hernia. *Pediatrics*, 99(6), 838-845.

Nield, T. A., Schrier, S., Ramos, A. D., Platzker, A. C., & Warburton, D. (1986). Unexpected hearing loss in high-risk infants. *Pediatrics*, 78(3), 417-422.

Nield, T. (2000). Neurodevelopmental outcome at 3.5 years of age in children treated with extracorporeal life support: Relationship to primary diagnosis. *The Journal of Pediatrics*, 136(3), 338-344.

Nijhuis-van der Sanden, M. W., van der Cammen-van Zijp, M. H., Janssen, A. J., Reuser, J. J., Mazer, P., van Heijst, A. F., et al. (2009). Motor performance in five-year-old extracorporeal membrane oxygenation survivors: a population-based study. *Crit Care*, 13(2), R47.

Nobuhara, K. K., Lund, D. P., Mitchell, J., Kharasch, V., & Wilson, J. M. (1996). Long-term outlook for survivors of congenital diaphragmatic hernia. *Clin Perinatol,* 23(4), 873-887.

Noori, S., Friedlich, P., Wong, P., Garingo, A., & Seri, I. (2007). Cardiovascular effects of sildenafil in neonates and infants with congenital diaphragmatic hernia and pulmonary hypertension. *Neonatology,* 91(2), 92-100.

Peetsold, M. G., Vonk-Noordegraaf, A., Heij, H. H., & Gemke, R. J. B. J. (2007). Pulmonary function and exercise testing in adult survivors of congenital diaphragmatic hernia. *Pediatric Pulmonology,* 42(4), 325-331.

Rasheed, A., Tindall, S., Cueny, D. L., Klein, M. D., & Delaney-Black, V. (2001). Neurodevelopmental outcome after congenital diaphragmatic hernia: Extracorporeal membrane oxygenation before and after surgery. *J Pediatr Surg,* 36(4), 539-544.

Reid, L. M. (1984). Lung growth in health and disease. *British Journal of Diseases of the Chest,* 78(2), 113-134.

Reiss, I., Schaible, T., van den Hout, L., Capolupo, I., Allegaert, K., van Heijst, A., et al. (2010). Standardized postnatal management of infants with congenital diaphragmatic hernia in Europe: the CDH EURO Consortium consensus. *Neonatology,* 98(4), 354-364.

Schwartz, I. P., Bernbaum, J. C., Rychik, J., Grunstein, M., D'Agostino, J., & Polin, R. A. (1999). Pulmonary hypertension in children following extracorporeal membrane oxygenation therapy and repair of congenital diaphragmatic hernia. *Journal of Perinatology,* 19(3), 220-226.

Steven, M. J., Fyfe, A. H. B., Raine, P. A. M., & Watt, I. (2007). Esophageal adenocarcinoma: a long-term complication of congenital diaphragmatic hernia? *Journal of Pediatric Surgery,* 42(7), e1-e3.

Su, W., Berry, M., Puligandla, P. S., Aspirot, A., Flageole, H., & Laberge, J. M. (2007). Predictors of gastroesophageal reflux in neonates with congenital diaphragmatic hernia. *J Pediatr Surg,* 42(10), 1639-1643.

Trachsel, D., Selvadurai, H., Bohn, D., Langer, J. C., & Coates, A. L. (2005). Long-term pulmonary morbidity in survivors of congenital diaphragmatic hernia. *Pediatr Pulmonol,* 39(5), 433-439.

Tracy, S., Estroff, J., Valim, C., Friedman, S., & Chen, C. (2010). Abnormal neuroimaging and neurodevelopmental findings in a cohort of antenatally diagnosed congenital diaphragmatic hernia survivors. *Journal of Pediatric Surgery,* 45(5), 958-965.

Tsao, K., Lally, P. A., & Lally, K. P. (2011). Minimally invasive repair of congenital diaphragmatic hernia. *Journal of Pediatric Surgery,* 46(6), 1158-1164.

Tulloh, R. (2009). Etiology, Diagnosis, and Pharmacologic Treatment of Pediatric Pulmonary Hypertension. *Pediatric Drugs,* 11(2), 115-128.

Vanamo, K., Rintala, R. J., Lindahl, H., & Louhimo, I. (1996). Long-term gastrointestinal morbidity in patients with congenital diaphragmatic defects. *Journal of Pediatric Surgery,* 31(4), 551-554.

Vanamo, K., Peltonen, J., Rintala, R., Lindahl, H., Jääskeläinen, J., & Louhimo, I. (1996). Chest wall and spinal deformities in adults with congenital diaphragmatic defects. *Journal of Pediatric Surgery,* 31(6), 851-854.

van den Hout, L., Reiss, I., Felix, J. F., Hop, W. C., Lally, P. A., Lally, K. P., et al. (2010). Risk factors for chronic lung disease and mortality in newborns with congenital diaphragmatic hernia. *Neonatology,* 98(4), 370-380.

van den Hout, L., Schaible, T., Cohen-Overbeek, T. E., Hop, W., Siemer, J., van de Ven, K., et al. (2011). Actual outcome in infants with congenital diaphragmatic hernia: the role of a standardized postnatal treatment protocol. *Fetal Diagnosis and Therapy,* 29(1), 55-63.

Van Meurs, K. P., Robbins, S. T., Reed, V. L., Karr, S. S., Wagner, A. E., Glass, P., et al. (1993). Congenital diaphragmatic hernia: long-term outcome in neonates treated with extracorporeal membrane oxygenation. *J Pediatr,* 122(6), 893-899.

Wilkens, H., Guth, A., König, J., Forestier, N., Cremers, B., Hennen, B., et al. (2001). Effect of Inhaled Iloprost Plus Oral Sildenafil in Patients With Primary Pulmonary Hypertension. *Circulation,* 104(11), 1218-1222.

Wischermann, A., Holschneider, A. M., & Hübner, U. (1995). Long-Term Follow-Up of Children with Diaphragmatic Hernia. *European Journal of Pediatric Surgery,* 5(01), 13,18.

Wright, J. C. E., Budd, J. L. S., Field, D. J., & Draper, E. S. (2011). Epidemiology and outcome of congenital diaphragmatic hernia: a 9-year experience. *Paediatric and Perinatal Epidemiology,* 25(2), 144-149.

11

Predictors of Mortality and Morbidity in Infants with CDH

Hany Aly[1] and Hesham Abdel-Hady[2]
[1]*The George Washington University*
[2]*Mansoura University,*
[1]*USA*
[2]*Egypt*

1. Introduction

Congenital diaphragmatic hernia (CDH) accounts for 8% of all major congenital anomalies with an incidence of 1 in 2000 to 4000 births (Doyle & K.P. Lally 2004). It is associated with significant mortality and morbidity (Abdullah et al., 2009). Survival data for CDH are conflicting; a few centers reported 82% to 93% survival rate (Javid et al., 2004; Grushka et al., 2009; Mettauer et al., 2009) while others had significantly less figures (54%-56%) (Colvin et al., 2005; Levison et al., 2006). This divergence in survival data has been attributed to case selection bias at single tertiary care institutions because as many as 35% of live-born infants with CDH do not survive to transport resulting in a hidden mortality for this condition (Harrison et al., 1978; Colvin et al.; 2005, V.K. Mah et al., 2009). Hidden mortality is referred to patients who die before surgery, either during gestation or shortly after birth, and thus are not reported by individual institutions (Harrison et al., 1994).

Neurodevelopmental impairment is the most important morbidity among CDH survivors, apart from respiratory complications (D'Agostino et al., 1995; Nobuhara et al., 1996; McGahren et al., 1997; Danzer et al., 2010). At 8-12 years of age, mean IQ is 85 (1 SD below age expectations) (Bouman et al. (2000), 45% have poor academic achievement, 50% are rated as having emotional and/or behavioral problems; by adolescent age, they have problems with sustained attention (39%) (Peetsold et al., 2009). Between 23-46% of CDH survivors demonstrate academic difficulties on standardized achievement measures, and more than half receive a formal diagnosis of specific learning disability, attention deficit hyperactivity disorder, or developmental disability. In almost one third of cases, difficulties are severe enough to require placement in a special education class (Frisk et al., 2011). Cognitive delay in this population could be attributed to perinatal and postnatal hypoxia and acidosis. Perioperative hypocapnia, related to aggressive ventilation, is also linked to executive dysfunction, behavioral problems, lowered intelligence, and poor intellectual achievement especially in mathematics (Frisk et al., 2011).

In this chapter we plan to provide a review on specific predictors for outcomes of CDH infants. These predictors include basic laboratory findings, prenatal and postnatal characteristics, type of medical support, and timing of surgical repair.

2. Prenatal identification and imaging (Table 1)

2.1 Prenatal identification

Prenatal identification of CDH does not necessarily improve the chance for postnatal survival. In fact, studies demonstrated a two to four fold increase in mortality among prenatally diagnosed CDH patients when compared with postnatally diagnosed patients (Skari et al., 2000). Although the reason behind this association is not clear, prenatal diagnosis of CDH may infer that the defect is larger with more displaced bowel and worse pulmonary hypoplasia (Laudy et al., 2003; Heling et al., 2005). Also, prenatal diagnosis has been associated with higher frequency of associated abnormalities, which may contribute to decreased survival of CDH children (Skari et al., 2002).

2.2 Lung to head ratio

The most commonly used method to assess fetal lung volume, and subsequent outcomes, is the measurement of lung area to head circumference ratio (LHR) with the use of 2-dimensional ultrasound (US) (Metkus et al., 1996; Sbragia et al., 2000; Laudy et al., 2003; Heling et al., 2005; Jani et al., 2006a; Hedrick et al., 2007; S.H. Yang et al., 2007; Sinha et al., 2009). Sonographic assessment of LHR usually takes place at 24–26 weeks gestation wherein lung is measured at the level of the four-chamber view of the heart. Minimum LHR measurements had a high inter- and intraobserver correlation (coefficients of 0.7 and 0.8, respectively) making it attractive (Ba'ath et al., 2007; Jani et al., 2007), and also proved to be related to survival (an inverse relation), independent of therapy. LHR <1.0 is usually not compatible with life, whereas LHR >1.4 is associated with virtually no mortality; LHR of 1 may be the survival 'threshold' (Jani et al., 2006a). A more frequently used indicator is the LHR of the contralateral lung (Metkus et al., 1996; Laudy et al., 2003), although some recent studies questioned its prognostic value (Heling et al., 2005; Arkovitz et al., 2007; Ba'ath et al., 2007).

Predictor	Factors associated with unfavorable outcomes
Ultrasound findings	Small lung to head ratio (LHR) at 24 weeks of gestation
	Discrepancy of observed to expected LHR for different gestational ages
	Abnormal Liver position
MRI findings	Small total fetal lung volume
	Dense lung fields, the ratio of the lung signal intensity to the spinal fluid signal intensity
Pulmonary vascular assessment	Small diameters of pulmonary artery and its branches
	Small flow volume and velocity
	Absent or shallow reactivity to maternal oxygen

Table 1. Fetal parameters used to predict CDH outcomes

Of note, LHR normally changes with advancing gestational age; therefore, a fixed cutoff, as initially proposed, can be misleading (Peralta et al., 2005; Ba'ath et al., 2007; Jani et al., 2007; Usui et al., 2007). Therefore, an observed-to-expected (O/E) LHR could be used regardless of the gestational age at which the study was done (Peralta et al., 2005; Jani et al., 2006b, Kilian et al., 2009). It is worth mentioning that the presence of abdominal viscera in the pleural space and contralateral displacement of the heart and mediastinum seem to play no role in the prognosis of CDH (Kalache et al., 2007).

2.3 Liver position

Liver position is the most significant and reproducible independent prenatal determinant of survival with liver herniation predictive of poor outcome (Albanese et al., 1998; Jani et al., 2006a; Hedrick et al., 2007). In a recent CDH series, newborns with the liver up had a mortality of approximately 55%, and 80% of CDH children born with intrathoracic liver position required extracorporeal membrane oxygenation (ECMO) (Hedrick et al., 2007). Intact discharge rates when the liver is down was shown to be 87%, while when the liver is up it ranged from 10%-47% (Kitano et al., 2011). As liver position is a predictor of severity, it is not surprising that liver herniation is not only predictive of survival but also predicts impaired neurodevelopmental outcome. Nearly 80% of CDH children with prenatally diagnosed liver herniation demonstrated borderline or delayed neurodevelopmental, neurocognitive, and/or psychomotor outcome (Danzer et al., 2010).

2.4 Total lung volume and signal intensity by MRI

Total fetal lung volume (TFLV) measured by magnetic resonance imaging (MRI) have also been reported to be useful in the prediction of pulmonary hypoplasia. Some studies report a significantly higher likelihood of death if the O/E TFLV were < 30-35% (Büsing et al., 2008; Cannie et al., 2008; Bonfils et al., 2006). This measurement is considered, to date, as the most accurate prognostic factor for survival of both left-sided and right-sided CDH (Gerards et al., 2008).

Studies using MRI signal intensity for fetuses with CDH showed both positive (Matsushita et al., 2008) and negative (Nishie et al., 2009; Balassy et al., 2010) data for prediction of survival prognosis. The ratio of the lung signal intensity to the spinal fluid signal intensity (L/SF) were significantly larger in survivors compared with deaths (0.82 vs 0.61, $P<0.05$). This ratio correlated with duration of tracheal intubation ($P<0.01$) (Terui et al., 2011).

2.5 Pulmonary vascular assessment

In addition to the severity of lung hypoplasia, the degree of pulmonary hypertension is equally important. Thus, in-utero assessment of lung vasculature seems another logical approach for predicting outcome. The branches, vessel diameters, flow velocimetry or flow volume can be measured using 2D or 3D ultrasound techniques (Suda et al., 2000; Sokol et al., 2006; Ruano et al. , 2007). Vascular indicators are more accurate as negative predictors, so that the absence of vascular abnormalities is a good sign but not vice versa (Fuke et al., 2003; Okazaki et al., 2008). There are limited preliminary data on the utility of testing the reactivity of fetal pulmonary vessels to maternal hyperoxygenation (Broth et al., 2002). Unfortunately, this test can only be done in late gestation.

3. Delivery hospital and need for transport

3.1 Location of delivery and neonatal transport

The quality of preoperative medical management can significantly impact outcomes of infants with CDH. This management includes resuscitation in the delivery room, medical stabilization in the early stages after birth, and the use of gentle ventilation to sustain adequate oxygenation while minimizing lung damage before surgery. Because these interventions require certain experiences and some technological resources such as extracorporeal membrane oxygenation (ECMO) that are not necessarily available in every birthing centers, it has been widely accepted to always deliver prenatally diagnosed CDH infants at high-risk perinatal centers. Maternal transfer is always safer than transfer of an unstable infant (Keshen et al., 1997; Sreenan et al., 2001; Boloker et al., 2002; Nasr et al., 2011). Location of delivery is a significant independent predictor for mortality, with an odds ratio (OR) of dying when outborn of 2.8 (Nasr et al., 2011). The thermal and hemodynamic instabilities that routinely occur during transport can be compromising to neonates; especially in the setting of CDH patients who have hypoplastic lungs and pulmonary hypertension. As up to one-third of infants with CDH may require ECMO therapy, some authors advocate delivery of infants with CDH in an ECMO center whenever possible (Sreenan et al., 2001). A recent study of a large database (Aly et al., 2010) demonstrated increased mortality and use of ECMO in CDH infants who utilized transport. Transported infants used more ECMO than non-transported ones (25% vs 15%; OR = 1.46) and had higher mortality after surgery (16% vs 13%; OR= 1.46). (Figure 1)

3.2 Hospital volume

A controversial area which has been highlighted is the difference in survival between infants treated in "high volume" and "low volume" centers. Recently studies showed high volume centers (treating more than five cases per year) to perform significantly better. These data support the paradigm of regionalized perinatal centers (Javid et al., 2004; Skari et al., 2004; Bucher et al., 2010).

Javid et al (2004) from the Canadian Pediatric Surgery Network identified 88 children treated at 14 children's hospitals over a period of 22 months; hospitals were grouped into low volume (<12 cases/yr) or high volume (>12 cases/yr). Low-volume hospitals had a significantly higher mortality compared with high volume hospitals (23% vs. 10%). A survey involving 13 pediatric surgical centers in Scandinavia have demonstrated a tendency towards better survival in the higher-volume centers (>5 cases/yr) (72.4%) than in the centers with lower volume (≤ 5 cases/yr) (58.7%), p =0.065 (Skari et al., 2004). Another study including 2203 infants from 37 children's hospitals categorized institutions into low-volume (< 6 cases/yr), medium-volume (6 –10 cases/yr), and high-volume (>10 cases/yr); compared with low-volume hospitals, medium-volume (aOR: 0.56, 95% CI: 0.32– 0.97, *P*= 0.05) and high-volume (aOR: 0.44, 95% CI: 0.23– 0.80, *P* < 0.01) hospitals had a significantly lower mortality (Bucher et al., 2010).

3.3 Mode of delivery

There is still some doubt about the preferred mode of delivery and the timing of delivery in case of a CDH pregnancy. Recent studies reported no significant differences in overall

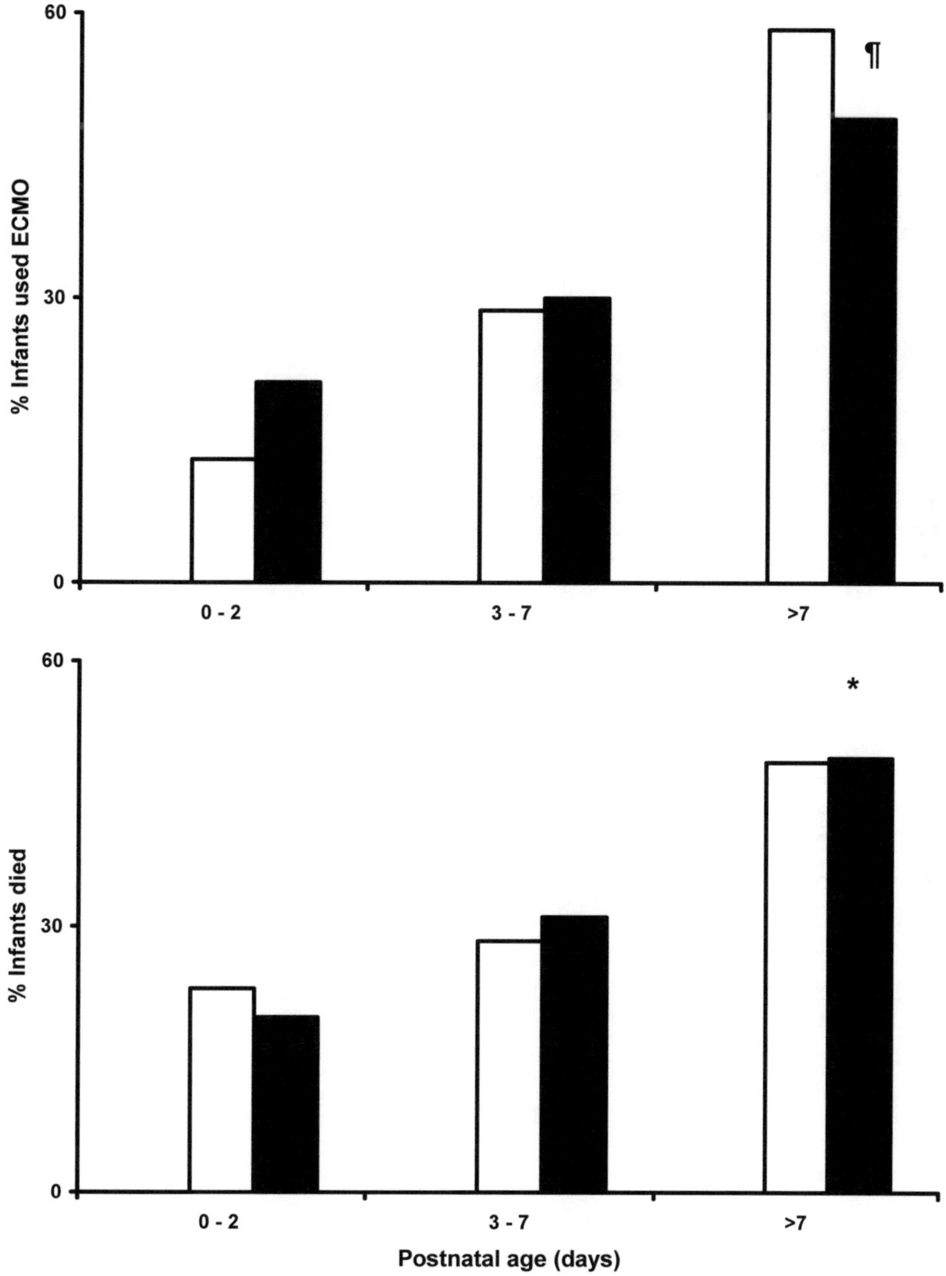

Fig. 1. Rates of mortality and use of ECMO in the study population stratified by date of surgery (Aly et al 2010)

The upper panel represents % of infants who used ECMO in the transported (■) and inborn (□) groups at the 3 different categories for age of operation. The lower panel represents % of infants who died in the transported (■) and inborn (□) groups at the 3 different categories for age of operation. ¶ * Risks for mortality and use of ECMO are increased when CDH repair was delayed > 7days (P <0.001) survival between patients born by spontaneous vaginal delivery, induced vaginal delivery and elective cesarean section (Frenckner et al., 2007; Stevens et al., 2009). Survival without the use of ECMO, however, was greater for patients born by elective cesarean section according to two studies (Bétrémieux et al., 2002; Frenckner et al., 2007).

4. Gestational age, birth weight, race and others (Table 2)

4.1 Gestational age and birth weight

Although outcomes for preterm infants are clearly worse than in the term infant, more than 50% of preterm infants still survived. Preterm infants with CDH remain a high-risk group. ECMO is of limited value in the extremely premature infant with CDH, however most preterm infants that live to undergo repair will survive. Survival decreases with decreasing gestational age. Prematurity should not be an independent factor in the treatment strategies of infants with CDH (Tsao et al., 2010).

A single study (Stevens et al., 2009) reported better outcomes in CDH infants when born at 37–38 weeks as compared to those born at 39–41 weeks gestation. There is no clear biological plausibility for such findings. Earlier data reported the opposite; that is better survival rates and a shorter duration of ECMO treatment in infants born at 40–42 weeks when compared to those born at 38–39 weeks gestation (Stevens et al., 2002). Therefore, the length of gestation should be determined based on an individualized approach.

Low birth weight has been identified as independent risk factors for poor outcomes (Keshen et al., 1997; Congenital Diaphragmatic Hernia Study Group, 2001; Stevens et al., 2002; Skarsgard et al., 2005; Haricharan et al., 2009; Bucher et al., 2010).

Predictor	Factors associated with unfavorable outcomes
Delivery location	Low hospital volume and inexperience with CDH
	Need for neonatal transport
Apgar score	Lower score at 5 minutes
Initial blood gases	Acidemia and hypoxemia
Gestational age	Prematurity
Birth weight	Lower birth weight

Table 2. Delivery location and perinatal predictors for CDH outcomes

4.2 Race and other factors

African Americans diagnosed with CDH have lower survival compared to Whites (W. Yang et al., 2006; Frencker et al., 2007; Stevens et al., 2009). Multivariate analysis confirmed that race was an independent predictor of mortality with African Americans and other race (not Hispanics) experiencing a greater than 50% excess mortality compared to Whites (Sola et al., 2010).

Environmental factors play an equal pivotal role in neurodevelopmental outcome of CDH. In fact, a low socio-economical status has been associated with a worse outcome. Stolar et al. (1995) found that low-level maternal education, as a potential surrogate for socio-economic status, significantly correlated with the incidence of abnormal neurocognitive outcome in

CDH children. It is obvious that advantaged environments can reduce the impact of medical risk factors, while poor environment and the lack of social support can amplify biological risk factors (Sameroff, 1998).

In infants with CDH, a prolonged neonatal hospitalization and the use of supplemental oxygen at the time of discharge are associated with a poorer neurological outcome (Nield et al., 2000; Cortes et al., 2005). These two conditions could reflect the role of the severity of the primary disease.

5. Apgar scores and early blood gases

5.1 Apgar scores

Poor Apgar score is an early marker for maladaptation to cardiopulmonary resuscitation. Poor Apgar scores at 1 and 5 minutes were associated with mortality (Chao et al., 2010). The CDH study group analyzed 2524 neonates undergoing repair and reported that the use of neonatal transport, gestational age less than 37 weeks, low birth weight (< 2 kg), prenatal diagnosis, associated major cardiac anomaly or chromosome anomaly, low 5-minute Apgar score, right-sided hernia, and agenesis of diaphragm or defects needing patch repair were significantly unfavorable factors for survival (Congenital Diaphragmatic Hernia Study Group et al., 2007). Another study identified three independent risk factors for mortality with CDH: low 5-minute Apgar score, prematurity, and air leak. Among these, 5-minute Apgar score was the strongest risk factor (Levison et al., 2006)

5.2 Arterial blood gases

Initial arterial blood gas (ABG) values have been linked to mortality since 1974 (Boix-Ochoa et al., 1974); since then ABG parameters have been used as indicators for the degree of pulmonary hypoplasia (Butt et al., 1992; Norden et al., 1994). Lower pH and lower PaO_2 in initial arterial blood gas (ABG) are associated with higher with mortality (Heiss & Clark, 1995; Chu et al., 2000; Chou et al., 2001; Haricharan et al., 2009; Chao et al., 2010).

Arterial PCO_2 is an accurate marker of the degree of lung hypoplasia and would explain the close association between severe hypercapnia (Pa CO_2 >60 mm Hg) and mortality (Bohn et al., 1984). However with the introduction of the concept for permissive hypercapnia to minimize ventilator-induced lung injury, tolerance to high $PaCO_2$ has become popular in neonates with CDH (Wung et al.,1985; Logan et al., 2007). Therefore, high $PaCO_2$ does not necessarily indicate lung hypoplasia but could rather indicate a more conservative ventilator management. Nowadays some centers are still reporting worse outcomes in CDH neonates if they had $PaCO_2$ values greater than 60 mm Hg before the initiation of ECMO (Haricharan et al., 2009).

6. Chest x-ray and echocardiographic findings

6.1 Chest x-ray

Currently it is believed that chest radiography serves to confirm the diagnosis of CDH, but does not predict outcome (Holt et al., 2004). Earlier attempts were made to correlate findings on plain-film chest radiography in CDH with rates of survival (Touloukian & Markowitz,

1984; Saifuddin & Arthur, 1993; Dimitriou et al., 2000). Positive predictors of survival included; ipsilateral lung aeration greater than 10%, contralateral lung aeration greater than 50%, mediastinum displaced by less than half the width (Donnelly et al., 1999). Poor signs included the presence of a contralateral pneumothorax, absence of contralateral aerated lung and an intrathoracic site for the stomach (Saifuddin & Arthur, 1993). Computer-assisted analysis of the lung area on the chest radiograph was thought to be a useful predictor postoperatively but not preoperatively (Dimitriou et al., 2000).

6.2 Echocardiography

A few studies focused on pulmonary artery size and pressure in CDH infants (Okazaki et al., 2008; Aggarwal et al., 2011a). When measured on the same day of birth, left and right pulmonary artery diameters and their ratios were significantly smaller among infants who died compared with those who survived (Aggarwal et al., 2011a). Persistent systemic or suprasystemic pulmonary artery pressure during the first 3 weeks of life was associated with decreased survival (Dillon et al., 2004). Calculating the ratio between the sum of the diameters of the 2 pulmonary arteries (measured at the hilus) and the diameter of the aorta (measured at the level of the diaphragm), could also be a good predictor of outcome in CDH (Suda et al., 2000).

The echocardiographic ratio of right ventricular systolic to diastolic duration was significantly higher in neonates with CDH, compared to term controls. Among infants with CDH, a ratio of 1.3 or greater was predictive of mortality (sensitivity= 93%and specificity= 62%) (Aggarwal et al., 2011b). Mortality was associated with the degree of impairment of global ventricular function and pulmonary hypertension (Aggarwal et al., 2011b).

The ratio of estimated pulmonary artery pressure to systemic pressure is helpful in assessing the severity of pulmonary hypertension. A ratio of 0.9 or greater preoperatively predicts mortality (sensitivity of 100% and specificity of 84%) (Al-Hathlol et al., 2011).

7. The diaphragmatic defect (Table 3)

7.1 Site of the diaphragmatic defect

Almost 20% of CDH is on the right-side and 1% is bilateral. Whether the site of the diaphragmatic defect is a significant factor in survival is controversial. Some studies reported higher mortality in right-sided CDH (Boix-Ochoa et al., 1974; Touloukian & Markowitz, 1984; Skari et al., 2000; Colvin et al., 2005; Jani et al, 2008; Chao et al., 2010; Schaible et al., 2012), others did not find statistical difference in mortality rate when compared with left-sided defects (Ontario Congenital Anomalies Study Group, 2004; J.E.Wright et al., 2010). Whether right-side CDH is associated with higher rates of malformations is also debatable (Skari, et al., 2000; Bedoyan et al., 2004; Hedrick et al., 2004). When the defect is bilateral, associated anomalies (Neville et al., 2003; Ninos et al., 2006) and mortality (Neville et al., 2003) are significantly increased.

7.2 Size of the diaphragmatic defect

Large hernia size—for which patch repair is a surrogate marker—strongly reduces overall survival as well as increases the risk of multiple adverse outcomes (D'Agostino et al., 1995;

McGahren et al., 1997; Cortes et al., 2005; Congenital Diaphragmatic Hernia Study Group et al., 2007; Danzer et al., 2010). Patch repair correlates with higher long-term morbidity, increased rate of gastroesophageal reflux and altered pulmonary function tests, especially in the first 6 months of life (Valfrè et al., 2011). A recent report from CDH Study Group found the size of the diaphragmatic defect to be the only independent risk factor associated with higher mortality rate (Congenital Diaphragmatic Hernia Study Group et al., 2007).

7.3 Associated malformations

The incidence of malformations in CDH infants is 33–50% (Fauza & J.M.Wilson, 1994; Colvin et al., 2005). Associated anomalies are very heterogeneous, but cardiovascular malformations are the most common (Zaiss et al., 2011). The presence of associated malformations increases mortality 4-6 folds (J.M.Wilson et al., 1997; Skari et al., 2000; Congenital Diaphragmatic Hernia Study Group, 2001; Stege et al., 2003; Colvin et al., 2005; Graziano & Congenital Diaphragmatic Hernia Study Group, 2005; W.Yang et al., 2006; J.E.Wright et al., 2010). Isolated CDH cases are more likely to survive and have lower morbidity than those occurring as part of a syndrome (Nobuhara et al., 1996; Doyle & K.P. Lally, 2004; Danzer et al., 2010).

Predictor	Factors associated with unfavorable outcomes
Diaphragmatic defect	Large size and need for patch
	Site of hernia (right vs. left) is controversial
	The presence of other associated anomalies
Medical management	Aggressive ventilation and hypocarbia are associated with morbidities
	Use of ECMO is associated with higher mortality and morbidities
	Prolonged hospitalization is a poor sign
	Oxygen supplementation at the time of hospital discharge is a poor sign

Table 3. Diaphragmatic defect and medical management as predictors of outcomes

8. Management strategy

8.1 Early, delayed, and very delayed surgical corrections

The timing of surgical repair has gradually shifted from emergent repair to delaying surgery until ventilatory and medical stabilization. The delay may range from several hours in stable patients up to several weeks in those subjected to ECMO therapy (Hosgor & Tibboel, 2004). However, surgery is generally performed at 24-96 hours (Nio et al., 1994), with the CDH study group noting a mean age at surgery of 73 hours for patients not treated with ECMO (Clark et al., 1998; Congenital Diaphragmatic Hernia Study Group, 2001).

It is important to note that surgical reduction of the hernia does not improve lung mechanics and may even temporarily decrease the compliance of the chest wall. This can be explained by increased abdominal pressure associated with reduction of the viscera into the small abdominal cavity (Sakai et al., 1987). Delayed surgery is theorized to provide additional time for remodeling of the pulmonary vasculature, leading to a more stable infant, who is better able to tolerate a postoperative decrease in compliance (Sakai et al., 1987; Boloker et al., 2002).

Although the evidence to support the delay in surgery is lacking (Skari et al., 2000; Moyer et al., 2002), logically it is safer not to operate on an infant during a transitional period of severe pulmonary hypertension and high oxygen demand. Two randomized trials showed no significant differences between early and late surgery, but risk stratification was difficult due to the small numbers (Nio et al., 1994; Frenckner et al., 1997). A recent study from United States National Database does not support a beneficiary effect for delaying surgical repair beyond 7 days. They have demonstrated no statistical difference in mortality, when comparing a group of babies operated before 3 days of life or between the ages of 3 to 7 days of life. However, when babies were operated after 7 days of life, their mortality and use of ECMO increased significantly. It is possible that infants who were not stabilized in the first 7 days of life before surgery had significant pulmonary hypertension and consequently had increased mortality. (Aly et al., 2010) (Figure 1)

We can reasonably conclude that the survival of infants with CDH is not affected by the duration of waiting but instead the rather specific physiologic parameters that need to be met before operating on CDH infants (Rozmiarek et al., 2004). These parameters include lower FiO2 requirement, minimal ventilator setting and absence of discrepancy between pre- and post-ductal saturations. Therefore, the European task force for CDH (CDH EURO Consortium) recommends performing surgical repair after physiological stabilization, defined as: mean arterial blood pressure normal for gestational age; preductal saturation range of 85% to 95% on fractional inspired oxygen less than 50%; plasma lactate concentration less than 3 mmol/l; and urine output more than 2 ml/kg/h (Reiss et al., 2010).

8.2 Ventilatory management

The most important facet in managing CDH infants is careful manipulation of ventilatory support. Given that pulmonary hypertension is ubiquitous in infants with CDH, reports of amelioration of ductal shunting in infants with persistent pulmonary hypertension prompted an era of aggressive hyperventilation (Drummond et al., 1981). Unfortunately, this was probably responsible for more mortality and morbidity than pulmonary hypoplasia and pulmonary hypertension combined. In 1995, Wung et al. (1995), demonstrated increased survival and decreased use of ECMO with the use of 'gentle ventilation', namely permissive hypercapnea, spontaneous respiration, avoidance of hyperventilation, avoidance of paralytic agents and continuous sedation infusion. Most centers now advocate prevention of ventilator-induced lung injury by tolerating hypercapnea while using low to moderate ventilator settings to achieve adequate pre-ductal oxygenation. Virtually all centers with survival over 80% employ this technique. The experience from Boston demonstrated that abandoning hyperventilation in favor of permissive hypercapnea resulted in an immediate 25% increase in survival (J.M.Wilson et al., 1997).

8.3 The use of extracorporeal membrane oxygenation (ECMO)

Roughly 50% of infants with high risk CDH are treated with ECMO (Breaux et al., 1991). Survival of CDH infants treated with ECMO is 40% (Aly et al., 2010). As an index of the degree of pulmonary hypoplasia, pre-ECMO pCO_2 is particularly predictive of survival in CDH infants requiring ECMO (Hoffman et al., 2011).

Infants who utilize ECMO are obviously those with a severe form of pulmonary hypertension, who would otherwise die if this technology was not available. These infants are shown to have greater use of diaphragmatic patches during repair and frequently undergo other procedures such as fundoplications and gastrostomy tube insertion (McGahren et al., 1997). Use of ECMO is associated with poorer neurological outcomes including; hearing deficits (Y. Sakurai et al., 1999, Lund et al., 1994; Nobuhara et al., 1996), brain abnormalities (Davenport et al., 1992; Lund et al., 1994), and developmental delay (Davenport et al., 1992; Nobuhara et al., 1996). However, as CDH survivors move through their school-age years, neurodevelopmental weaknesses become more apparent.

Between 10%-30% of patients treated with ECMO, including CDH-survivors, have neurological deficits (Towne et al., 1985; Glass et al., 1989; Schumacher et al., 1991). Among ECMO survivors, the diagnosis of CDH does not independently contribute to neurological risk (Stolar et al. 1995) although CDH infants are more unstable and have more complications while on ECMO (Stolar et al., 1995). The rate of adverse neurologic sequelae is lower when ECMO used with venovenous cannulation (Dimmitt et al., 2001; Kugelman et al., 2003). Therefore, ECMO improved survival in infants with CDH without long-term benefit (Morini et al., 2006).

The duration of ECMO has a substantial impact on survival. Beyond two weeks of ECMO support, survival decreases significantly (Tiruvoipati et al., 2007; Seetharamaiah et al., 2009). This could be related to increased renal, hematological, and CNS complications (Stevens et al. 2002). However, even after controlling for complications, duration of ECMO independently affected survival (Haricharan et al., 2009). Prolonged ECMO is a marker for severe pulmonary hypoplasia with its associated ventilation and oxygenation issues. Also, prolonged ECMO causes amplification of inflammatory response that may lead to severe edema and progressive organ dysfunction (Radhakrishnan & Cox, 2005).

9. Conclusion

Despite advances in neonatal care and surgeries, mortality and morbidity of infants with CDH are significant. There are multiple predictors for adverse outcomes in this population. Fetal lung volume can be measured via ultrasound or MRI. Early postnatal indicators for the severity of the disease include Apgar score at 5 minutes and early blood gas parameters. Delivery at a regional perinatal center without subsequent need for transport is favorable. Gentile ventilation and delaying surgery until physiological stabilization are associated with better outcomes. The use of ECMO is indicative of severe pulmonary hypertension and hemodynamic instability that are associated with worse outcomes.

10. References

Abdullah, F.; Zhang, Y.; Sciortino, C.; Camp, M.; Gabre-Kidan, A.; Price, M.R. & Chang, D.C. (2009). Congenital diaphragmatic hernia: outcome review of 2,173 surgical repairs in US infants. *Pediatr Surg Int*, Vol. 25, No. 12, (December 2009), pp. 1059-1064, ISSN: 0179-0358

Aggarwal, S.; Stockmann, P.T.; Klein, M.D. & Natarajan, G. (2011a). The right ventricular systolic to diastolic duration ratio: a simple prognostic marker in congenital diaphragmatic hernia?. *Acta Paediatr*, Vol. 100, No. 10, (October 2011), pp. 1315-1318, ISSN: 0803-5253

Aggarwal, S.; Stockmann, P.; Klein, M.D. & Natarajan, G. (2011b). Echocardiographic measures of ventricular function and pulmonary artery size: prognostic markers of congenital diaphragmatic hernia? *J Perinatol*, Vol. 31, No. 8, (August 2011), pp. 561-566, ISSN: 0743-8346

Albanese, C.T.; Lopoo, J.; Goldstein, R.B.; Filly, R.A.; Feldstein, V.A.; Calen, P.W.; Jennings, R.W.; Farrell, J.A. & Harrison, M.R. (1998). Fetal liver position and perinatal outcome for congenital diaphragmatic hernia. *Prenat Diagn*, Vol. 18, No. 11, (November 1998), pp.1138–1142, ISSN: 0197-3851

Al-Hathlol, K.; Elmahdy, H.; Nawaz, S.; Ali, I.; Tawakol, H.; Tawil, K. & Al-Saif, S. (2011). Perioperative course of pulmonary hypertension in infants with congenital diaphragmatic hernia: impact on outcome following successful repair. *J Pediatr Surg*, Vol. 46, No. 4, (April, 2011), pp. 625–629, ISSN: 0022-3468

Aly, H.; Bianco-Batlles, D.; Mohamed, M.A. & Hammad, T.A. (2010). Mortality in infants with congenital diaphragmatic hernia: a study of the United States National Database. *J Perinatol*, Vol. 30, No. 8, (August 2010), pp.553–557, ISSN: 0743-8346

Arkovitz, M.S.; Russo, M.; Devine, P.; Budhorick, N. & Stolar, C.J. (2007). Fetal lung-head ratio is not related to outcome for antenatal diagnosed congenital diaphragmatic hernia. *J Pediatr Surg*, Vol. 42, No. 1, (January 2007), pp. 107–110, ISSN: 0022-3468

Ba'ath, M.E.; Jesudason, E.C. & Losty, P.D. (2007). How useful is the lung-to-head ratio in predicting outcome in the fetus with congenital diaphragmatic hernia? A systematic review and meta-analysis. *Ultrasound Obstet Gynecol*, Vol. 30, No. 6, (November 2007), pp. 897-906, ISSN: 0960-7692

Balassy, C.; Kasprian, G.; Brugger, P.C.; Weber, M.; Csapo, B.; Herold, C. & Prayer D. (2010). Assessment of lung development in isolated congenital diaphragmatic hernia using signal intensity ratios on fetal MR imaging. *Eur Radiol*, Vol. 20, No. 4, (April 2010), pp. 829–837, ISSN: 1613-3749

Bedoyan, J.K.; Blackwell, S.C.; Treadwell, M.C.; Johnson, A. & Klein, M.D. (2004). Congenital diaphragmatic hernia: associated anomalies and antenatal diagnosis. *Pediatr Surg Int*, Vol. 20, No.3, (March 2004), pp. 170–176, ISSN: 0179-0358

Bétrémieux, P.; Lionnais, S.; Beuchée, A.; Pladys, P.; Le Bouar, G.; Pasquier, L.; Loeuillet-Olivo, L.; Azzis, O.; Milon, J.; Wodey, E.; Frémond, B.; Odent, S. & Poulain, P. (2002). Perinatal management and outcome of prenatally diagnosed congenital diaphragmatic hernia: a 19952000 series in Rennes University Hospital. *Prenat Diagn*, Vol. 22, No. 11, (November 2002), pp. 988-994, ISSN: 0197-3851

Bohn, D.J.; James, I.; Filler, R.M.; Ein, S.H.; Wesson, D.E.; Shandling, B.; Stephens, C.; Barker, G.A. (1984). The relationship between PaCO2 and ventilation parameters in predicting survival in congenital diaphragmatic hernia. *J Pediatr Surg*, Vol. 19, No. 9, (December 1984), pp. 666-671, ISSN: 0022-3468

Boix-Ochoa, J.; Peguero, G.; Seijo, G.; Natal, A. & Canals, J. (1974). Acid-base balance and blood gases in prognosis and therapy of congenital diaphragmatic hernia. *J Pediatr Surg*, Vol. 9, No. 1, (February 1974), pp. 49–57, ISSN: 0022-3468

Boloker, J.; Bateman, D.A.; Wung, J.T. & Stolar CJ. (2002). Congenital diaphragmatic hernia in 120 infants treated consecutively with permissive hypercapnea/spontaneous respiration/elective repair. *J Pediatr Surg,* Vol. 37, No. 3, (March 2002), pp. 357-366, ISSN: 0022-3468

Bonfils, M.; Emeriaud, G.; Durand, C.; Brancato, S.; Nugues, F.; Jouk, P.S.; Wroblewski, I. & Debillon, T. (2006). Fetal lung volume in congenital diaphragmatic hernia. *Arch Dis Child Fetal Neonatal Ed,* Vol. 91, No. 5, (September 2006), pp. F363–F364, ISSN: 1359-2998

Bouman, N.H.; Koot, H.M.; Tibboel, D. & Hazebroek, F.W. (2000). Children with congenital diaphragmatic hernia are at risk for lower levels of cognitive functioning and increased emotional and behavioral problems. *Eur J Pediatr Surg,* Vol. 10, No. 1, (February 2000), pp. 3–7, ISSN: 0022-3468

Bucher, B.T.; Guth, R.M.; Saito, J.M.; Najaf, T. & Warner, B.W. (2010). Impact of Hospital volume on in-hospital mortality of infants undergoing repair of congenital diaphragmatic hernia. *Ann Surg,* Vol. 252, No. 4, (October 2010), pp. 635–642, ISSN: 0003-4932

Butt, W.; Taylor, B. & Shann, F. (1992). Mortality prediction in infants with congenital diaphragmatic hernia: potential criteria for ECMO. *Anaesth Intensive Care,* Vol. 20, No. 4, (November 1992), pp.439-442, ISSN: 0310-057X

Breaux, C.W. Jr.; Rouse, T.M.; Cain, W.S. & Georgeson, K.E. (1991). Improvement in survival of patients with congenital diaphragmatic hernia utilizing a strategy of delayed repair after medical and/or extracorporeal membrane oxygenation stabilization. *J Pediatr Surg,* Vol. 26, No. 3, pp. 333–336, ISSN: 0022-3468

Broth, R.E.; Wood, D.C.; Rasanen, J.; Rasanen, J.; Sabogal, J.C.; Komwilaisak, R.; Weiner, S. & Berghella, V. (2002). Prediction of lethal pulmonary hypoplasia: the hyperoxygenation test for pulmonary artery reactivity. *Am J Obstet Gynecol,* Vol. 187, No. 4, (2002), pp. 940–945, ISSN: 0002-9378

Büsing, K.A.; Kilian, A.K.; Schaible, T.; Endler, C.; Schaffelder, R. & Neff, K.W. (2008). MR relative fetal lung volume in congenital diaphragmatic hernia: survival and need for extracorporeal membrane oxygenation. *Radiology,* Vol. 248, No. 1, (July 2008) pp. 240-246, ISSN: 0033-8419

Cannie, M.; Jani, J.; Meersschaert, J.; Allegaert, K.; Done', E.; Marchal, G. & Deprest, J. & Dymarkowski, S. (2008). Prenatal prediction of survival in isolated diaphragmatic hernia using observed to expected total fetal lung volume determined by magnetic resonance imaging based on either gestational age or fetal body volume. *Ultrasound Obstet Gynecol,* Vol. 32, No. 5, (October 2008), pp. 633-639, ISSN: 0960-7692

Chao, P.; Huang, C.; Liu, C.; Chung, M.; Chen, C.; Chen, F.; Ou-Yang, M. & Huang, H. (2010). Congenital Diaphragmatic Hernia in the Neonatal Period: Review of 21 Years' Experience. *Pediatr Neonatol,* Vol. 51, No. 2, (April 2010), pp. 97–102, ISSN: 1875-9572

Chou, H.C.; Tang, J.R.; Lai, H.S.; Tsao, P.N. & Yau, K.I. (2001). Prognostic indicators of survival in infants with congenital diaphragmatic hernia. *J Formos Med Assoc,* Vol. 100, No. 3, (March 2001), pp. 173–175, ISSN: 0929-6646

Chu, S.M.; Hsieh, W.S.; Lin, J.N.; Yang, P.H.; Fu, R.H. & Kuo, C.Y. (2000). Treatment and outcome of congenital diaphragmatic hernia. *J Formos Med Assoc,* Vol. 99, No. 11, (November 2000), pp. 844–847, ISSN: 0929-6646

Clark, R.H.; Hardin, W.D.; Hirshl, R.B.; Jaksic, T; Lally, K.P.; Langham, M.R.Jr. & Wilson, J.M. (1998). Current surgical management of congenital diaphragmatic hernia: A report from the Congenital Diaphragmatic Hernia Study Group. *J Pediatr Surg*, Vol. 33, No. 7, (July 1998), pp. 1004-1009, ISSN: 0022-3468

Colvin, J.; Bower, C.; Dickinson, J.E. & Sokol, J. (2005). Outcomes of congenital diaphragmatic hernia: a population-based study in Western Australia. *Pediatrics*, Vol. 117, No. 5, (May 2005), pp. 356-363, ISSN: 0031-4005

Congenital Diaphragmatic Hernia Study Group. (2001). Estimating disease severity of congenital diaphragmatic hernia in the first 5 minutes of life. The Congenital Diaphragmatic Hernia Study Group. *J Pediatr Surg*, Vol. 36, No. 1, (January 2001), pp. 141-145, ISSN: 0022-3468

Congenital Diaphragmatic Hernia Study Group; Lally, K.P.; Lally, P.A.; Lasky, R.E.; Tibboel, D.; Jaksic, T.; Wilson, J.M.; Frenckner, B.; Van Meurs, K.P.; Bohn, D.J.; Davis, C.F.; Hirschl, R.B. (2007). Defect size determines survival in infants with congenital diaphragmatic hernia. *Pediatrics*, Vol. 120, No. 3, (September 2007), pp. e651–e657, ISSN: 0031-4005

Cortes, R.A.; Keller, R.L.; Townsend, T.; Harrison, M.R.; Farmer, D.L.; Lee, H.; Piecuch, R.E.; Leonard, C.H.; Hetherton, M.; Bisgaard, R. & Nobuhara, K.K. (2005). Survival of severe congenital diaphragmatic hernia has morbid consequences. *J Pediatr Surg*, Vol. 40, No. 1, (January 2005), pp. 36–45, ISSN: 0022-3468

D'Agostino, J.A.; Bernbaum, J.C.; Gerdes, M.; Schwartz, I.P.; Coburn, C.E.; Hirschl, R.B.; Baumgart, S & Polin, R.A. (1995). Outcome for infants with congenital diaphragmatic hernia requiring extracorporeal membrane oxygenation: the first year. *J Pediatr Surg*, Vol. 30, No. 1, (January 1995), pp. 10-15, ISSN: 0022-3468

Danzer, E.; Gerdes, M.; Bernbaum, J.; D'Agostino, J.; Bebbington, M.W.; Siegle, J.; Hoffman, C.; Rintoul, N.E.; Flake, A.W.; Adzick, N.S. & Hedrick, H.L. (2010). Neurodevelopmental outcome of infants with congenital diaphragmatic hernia prospectively enrolled in an interdisciplinary follow-up program. *J Pediatr Surg*, Vol. 45, No. 9, (Septmber 2010), pp. 1759–1766, ISSN: 0022-3468

Davenport, M.; Rivlin, E.; D'Souza, S.W. & Bianchi, A. (1992). Delayed surgery for congenital diaphragmatic hernia: neurodevelopmental outcome in later childhood. *Arch Dis Child*, Vol. 67, No. 11, (November 1992), pp. 1353–1356, ISSN: 0003-9888

Dillon, P.W.; Cilley, R.E.; Mauger, D.; Zachary, C. & Meier, A. (2004). The relationship of pulmonary artery pressure and survival in congenital diaphragmatic hernia. *J Pediatr Surg*, Vol. 39, No. 3, (March 2004), pp. 307–312, ISSN: 0022-3468

Dimitriou, G.; Greenough, A.; Davenport, M. & Nicolaides K. (2000). Prediction of outcome by compute–assisted analysis of lung area on the chest radiograph of infants with congenital diaphragmatic hernia. *J Pediatr Surg*, Vol. 35, No. 3, (March 2000), pp. 489–493, ISSN: 0022-3468

Dimmitt, R.A.; Moss, R.L.; Rhine, W.D.; Benitz, W.E.; Henry, M.C. & Vanmeurs, K.P. (2001). Venoarterial versus venovenous extracorporeal membrane oxygenation in congenital diaphragmatic hernia: the extracorporeal life support organization registry, 1990–1999. *J Pediatr Surg*, Vol. 36, No. 8, (December 2001), pp. 1199–1204, ISSN: 0022-3468

Donnelly, L.; Sakurai, T.; Klosterman, L.; Delong, D.M. & Strife, J.L. (1999) Correlation between findings on chest radiography and survival in neonates with congenital diaphragmatic hernia. *Am J Roentgenol*, Vol. 173, No. 6, (December 1999), pp. 1589–1593, ISSN: 0361-803X

Doyle, N. & Lally, K.P. (2004). The CDH Study Group and advances in the clinical care of the patient with congenital diaphragmatic hernia. *Semin Perinatol,* Vol. 28, No. 3, (June 2004), pp. 174-184, ISSN 0146-0005

Drummond, W.H.; Gregory, G.A.; Heymann, M.A. & Phibbs, R.A. (1981). The independent effects of hyperventilation, tolazoline, and dopamine on infants with persistent pulmonary hypertension. *J Pediatr,* Vol. 98, No. 4, (April 1981), pp. 603-611, ISSN: 0022-3476

Fauza, D.O. & Wilson, J.M. (1994). Congenital diaphragmatic hernia and associated anomalies: their incidence, identification, and impact on prognosis. *J Pediatr Surg,* Vol. 29, No. 8, (August 1994), pp. 1113–1117, ISSN: 0022-3468

Frenckner, B.; Ehren, H.; Granholm, T.; Linden, V. & Palmer, K. (1997). Improved results in patients who have congenital diaphragmatic hernia using preoperative stabilization, extracorporeal membrane oxygenation, and delayed surgery. *J Pediatr Surg,* Vol. 32, No. 8, (August 1997), pp. 1185-1189, ISSN: 0022-3468

Frenckner, B.P.; Lally, P.A.; Hintz, S.R.; Lally, K.P. & Congenital Diaphragmatic Hernia Study Group. (2007). Prenatal diagnosis of congenital diaphragmatic hernia: how should the babies be delivered? *J Pediatr Surg,* Vol. 42, No. 9, (September 2007), pp. 1533-1538, ISSN: 0022-3468

Frisk, V.; Jakobson, L.S.; Unger, S.; Trachsel, D. & O'Brien, K. (2011). Long-term neurodevelopmental outcomes of congenital diaphragmatic hernia survivors not treated with extracorporeal membrane oxygenation. *J Pediatr Surg,* Vol. 46, No. 7, (July 2011), pp. 1309-1318, ISSN: 0022-3468

Fuke, S.; Kanzaki, T.; Mu, J.; Wasada, K.; Takemura, M.; Mitsuda, N. & Murata, Y. (2003). Antenatal prediction of pulmonary hypoplasia by acceleration time/ejection time ratio of fetal pulmonary arteries by Doppler blood flow velocimetry. *Am J Obstet Gynecol,* Vol. 188, No. 1 , (January 2003), pp. 228–233, ISSN: 0002-9378

Gerards, F.A.; Twisk, J.W.; Tibboel, D. & van Vugt, J.M. (2008). Congenital diaphragmatic hernia: 2D lung area and 3D lung volume measurements of the contralateral lung to predict postnatal outcome. *Fetal Diagn Ther,* Vol. 24, No. 3, (September 2008), pp. 271–276, ISSN: 1015-3837

Glass, P.; Miller, M. & Short, B.L. (1989). Morbidity for survivors of extracorporal membrane oxygenation: neurodevelopmental outcome at 1 year of age. *Pediatrics,* Vol. 83, No. 1, (January 1989), pp. 72–78, ISSN: 0031-4005

Graziano, J.N. & Congenital Diaphragmatic Hernia Study Group. (2005). Cardiac anomalies in patients with congenital diaphragmatic hernia and their prognosis: a report from the Congenital Diaphragmatic Hernia Study Group. *J Pediatr Surg,* Vol. 40, No. 6, (June 2005), pp. 1045-1049, ISSN: 0022-3468

Grushka, J.R.; Laberge, J.M.; Puligandla, P.; Skarsgard, E.D. & Canadian Pediatric Surgery Network. (2009). Effect of hospital case volume on outcome in congenital diaphragmatic hernia: the experience of the Canadian Pediatric Surgery Network. *J Pediatr Surg,* Vol. 44, No. 5, (May 2009), pp. 873-876, ISSN: 0022-3468

Haricharan, R.N.; Barnhart, D.C.; Cheng, H. & Delzell, E. (2009). Identifying neonates at a very high risk for mortality among children with congenital diaphragmatic hernia managed with extracorporeal membrane oxygenation. *J Pediatr Surg,* Vol. 44, No. 1, (January 2009), pp. 87–93, ISSN: 0022-3468

Harrison, M.R.; Bjordal, R.I.; Langmark, F. & Knutrud O. (1978). Congenital diaphragmatic hernia: The hidden mortality. *J Pediatr Surg,* Vol. 13, No. 3, (June 1978), pp. 227-230, ISSN: 0022-3468

Harrison, M.R.; Adzick, S.; Estes, J.M. & Howell, L.J. (1994). A prospective study of the outcome for fetuses with diaphragmatic hernia. *JAMA,* Vol. 271, No. 5, (February 1994), pp. 382-384, ISSN: 0098-7484

Hedrick, H.L.; Crombleholme, T.M.; Flake, A.W.; Nance, M.L.; von Allmen, D.; Howell, L.J., Johnson, M.P.; Wilson, R.D. & Adzick, N.S. (2004). Right congenital diaphragmatic hernia: prenatal assessment and outcome. *J Pediatr Surg,* Vol. 39, No. 3, (March 2004), pp. 319–323, ISSN: 0022-3468

Hedrick, H.L.; Danzer, E.; Merchant, A.; Bebbington, M.W.; Zhao, H.; Flake, A.W.; Johnson, M.P.; Liechty, K.W.; Howell, L.J.; Wilson, R.D. & Adzick NS. (2007). Liver position and lung-to-head ratio for prediction of extracorporeal membrane oxygenation and survival in isolated left congenital diaphragmatic hernia. *Am J Obstet Gynecol,* Vol. 197, No. 4, (October 2007), 422.e1-4, ISSN: 0002-9378

Heiss, K.F. & Clark, R.H. (1995). Prediction of mortality in neonates with congenital diaphragmatic hernia treated with extracorporeal membrane oxygenation. *Crit Care Med,* Vol. 23, No. 11, (November 1995), pp. 1915-1919, ISSN: 0090-3493

Heling, K.S., Wauer, R.R., Hammer, H., Bollmann, R. & Chaoui, R. (2005). Reliability of the lung-to-head ratio in predicting outcome and neonatal ventilation parameters in fetuses with congenital diaphragmatic hernia. *Ultrasound Obstet Gynecol,* Vol. 25, No. 2, (February 2005), pp. 112–118, ISSN: 0960-7692

Hoffman, S.B.; Massaro, A.N.; Gingalewski, C. & Short, B.L. (2011). Survival in congenital diaphragmatic hernia: use of predictive equations in the ECMO population. *Neonatology,* Vol. 99, No. 4, (November 2011), pp. 258–265, ISSN: 1661-7800

Holt, P.D.; Arkovitz, M.S.; Berdon, W.E. & Stolar, C.J. (2004). Newborns with diaphragmatic hernia: initial chest radiography does not have a role in predicting clinical outcome. *Pediatr Radiol,* Vol. 34, No. 6, (June 2004), pp. 462–464, ISSN: 0301-0449

Hosgor, M. & Tibboel, D. (2004). Congenital diaphragmatic hernia; many questions, few answers. *Paediatr Respir Rev,* Vol. 5, No. Suppl A, (2004), pp. S277–S282, ISSN: 1526-0542

Jani, J., Keller; R.L.; Benachi, A.; Nicolaides, K.H.; Favre, R.; Gratacos, E.; Laudy, J.; Eisenberg, V.; Eggink, A.; Vaast, P.; Deprest, J. & Antenatal-CDH-Registry Group. (2006a). Prenatal prediction of survival in isolated left-sided diaphragmatic hernia. *Ultrasound Obstet Gynecol,* Vol. 27, No. 1, (January 2006), pp. 18-22, ISSN: 0960-7692

Jani, J.; Peralta, C.F.; Van Schoubroeck, D.; Deprest, J. & Nicolaides, K.H. (2006b). Relationship between lung-to-head ratio and lung volume in normal fetuses and fetuses with diaphragmatic hernia. *Ultrasound Obstet Gynecol,* Vol. 25, No. 5, (May 2006), pp. 545-550, ISSN: 0960-7692

Jani, J.; Nicolaides, K.H.; Keller, R.L.; Benachi, A.; Peralta, C.F.; Favre, R.; Moreno, O.; Tibboel, D.; Lipitz, S.; Eggink, A.; Vaast, P.; Allegaert, K.; Harrison, M.; Deprest, J. & Antenatal-CDH-Registry Group. (2007). Observed to expected lung area to head circumference ratio in the prediction of survival in fetuses with isolated diaphragmatic hernia. *Ultrasound Obstet Gynecol,* Vol. 30, No. 1, (July 2007), pp. 67-71, ISSN: 0960-7692

Jani, J.; Nicolaides, K.H.; Benachi, A.; Moreno, O.; Favre, R.; Gratacos, E. & Deprest, J. (2008). Timing of lung size assessment using the observed to expected lung area to head circumference ratio in the prediction of postnatal survival in fetuses with isolated diaphragmatic hernia. *Ultrasound Obstet Gynecol,* Vol. 31, No. 1, (January 2008), 37-40, ISSN: 0960-7692

Javid, P.J.; Jaksic, T.; Skarsgard, E.D.; Lee, S. & Canadian Neonatal Network. (2004). Survival rate in congenital diaphragmatic hernia: the experience of the Canadian Neonatal Network. *J Pediatr Surg,* Vol. 39, No. 5, (May 2004), pp. 657-660, ISSN: 0022-3468

Kalache, K.D.; Mkhitaryan, M.; Bamberg, C.; Roehr, C.C.; Wauer, R.; Mau, H. & Bollmann R. (2007). Isolated left-sided congenital diaphragmatic hernia: cardiac axis and displacement before fetal viability has no role in predicting postnatal outcome. *Prenat Diagn,* Vol. 27, No. 4, (April 2007); 27, pp. 322–326, ISSN: 0197-3851

Keshen, T.H.; Gursoy, M.; Shew, S.B.; Smith, E.O.; Miller, R.G.; Wearden, M.E., Moise, A.A. & Jaksic, T. (1997). Does extracorporeal membrane oxygenation benefit neonates with congenital diaphragmatic hernia? Application of a predictive equation. *J Pediatr Surg,* Vol. 32 , No. 6, (June 1997), pp. 818-822, ISSN: 0022-3468

Kilian, A.K.; Schaible, T.; Hofmann, V.; Brade, J.; Neff, K.W. & Büsing, K.A. (2009). Congenital diaphragmatic hernia: predictive value of MRI relative lung-to head ratio compared with MRI fetal lung volume and sonographic lung-to-head ratio. *Am J Roentgenol,* Vol. 192, No. 1, (January 2009), pp. 153-158, ISSN: 0361-803X

Kitano, Y.; Okuyama, H.; Saito, M.; Usui, N.; Morikawa, N.; Masumoto, K.; Takayasu, H.; Nakamura, T.; Ishikawa, H.; Kawataki, M.; Hayashi, S., Inamura, N.; Nose, K.; Sago, H. (2011). Re-evaluation of stomach position as a simple prognostic factor in fetal left congenital diaphragmatic hernia: a multicenter survey in Japan. *Ultrasound Obstet Gynecol,* Vol. 37, No. 3, (March 2011), pp. 277–282, ISSN: 0960-7692

Kugelman, A.; Gangitano, E.; Pincros, J.; Tantivit, P.; Taschuk, R. & Durand, M. (2003). Venovenous versus venoarterial extracorporeal membrane oxygenation in congenital diaphragmatic hernia. *J Pediatr Surg,* Vol. 38, No. 8, (August 2003), pp. 1131–1136, ISSN: 0022-3468

Laudy, J.A.; Van Gucht, M.; Van Dooren, M.F.; Wladimiroff, J.W. & Tibboel, D. (2003). Congenital diaphragmatic hernia: an evaluation of the prognostic value of the lung-to-head ratio and other prenatal parameters. *Prenat Diagn,* Vol. 23, No. 8, (August 2003), pp. 634–639, ISSN: 0197-3851

Levison, J.; Halliday, R.; Holland, A.J.; Walker, K.; Williams, G.; Shi, E.; Badawi, N. & Neonatal Intensive Care Units Study of the NSW Pregnancy and Newborn Services Network. (2006). A population-based study of congenital diaphragmatic hernia outcome in New South Wales and the Australian Capital Territory, Australia, 1992−2001. *J Pediatr Surg,* Vol. 41, No. 6, (June 2006), pp. 1049−1053, ISSN: 0022-3468

Logan, J.W., Rice, H.E., Goldberg, R.N., Cotten CM. (2007). Congenital diaphragmatic hernia: a systematic review and summary of best-evidence practice strategies. *J Perinatol,* Vol. 27, No. 9, (September 2007), pp. 535-549, ISSN: 0743-8346

Lund, D.P.; Mitchell, J.; Kharasch, V.; Quigley, S.; Kuehn M. & Wilson, J.M. (1994). Congenital diaphragmatic hernia: the hidden morbidity. *J Pediatr Surg,* Vol. 29, No. 2 (February 1994), pp. 258–262, ISSN: 0022-3468

Mah, V.K.; Zamakhshary, M.; Mah, D.Y.; Cameron, B.; Bass, J., Bohn, D.; Scott, L., Himidan, S; Walker, M. & Kim PC. (2009). Absolute vs relative improvements in congenital diaphragmatic hernia survival: what happened to "hidden mortality. *J Pediatr Surg,* Vol. 44, No. 5, (May 2009), pp. 877-882, ISSN: 0022-3468

Matsushita, M.; Ishii, K.; Tamura, M.; Takahashi, Y.; Kamura, T.; Takakuwa, K. &Tanaka, K. (2008). Perinatal magnetic resonance fetal lung volumetry and fetal lung-to-liver signal intensity ratio for predicting short outcome in isolated congenital diaphragmatic hernia and cystic adenomatoid malformation of the lung. *J Obstet Gynaecol Res,* Vol 34, No. 2, (April 2008), pp. 162–167, ISSN: 1341-8076

McGahren, E.D.; Mallik, K. & Rodgers, B.M. (1997). Neurological outcome is diminished in survivors of congenital diaphragmatic hernia requiring extracorporeal membrane oxygenation. *J Pediatr Surg,* Vol. 32, No. 8, (August 1997), pp. 1216-1220, ISSN: 0022-3468

Metkus, A.P.; Filly, R.A.; Stringer, M.D.; Harrison, M.R. & Adzick, N.S. (1996). Sonographic predictors of survival in fetal diaphragmatic hernia. *J Pediatr Surg,* Vol. 31, No. 1, (January 1996), pp. 148-152, ISSN: 0022-3468

Mettauer, N.L.; Pierce, C.M.; Cassidy, J.V.; Kiely, E.M. & Petros, A.J. (2009). One-year survival in congenital diaphragmatic hernia, 1995-2006. *Arch Dis Child,* Vol. 94, No. 5, (May 2009), pp. 407, ISSN: 0003-9888

Morini, F.; Goldman, A. & Pierro, A. (2006). Extracorporeal membrane oxygenation in infants with congenital diaphragmatic hernia: a systematic review of the evidence. *Eur J Pediatr Surg,* Vol. 16, No. 6, (December 2006), pp. 385-391, ISSN: 0022-3468

Moyer, V.; Moya, F.; Tibboel, R.; Losty, P.; Nagaya, M. & Lally, K.P. (2002). Late versus early surgical correction for congenital diaphragmatic hernia in newborn infants. *Cochrane Database Syst Rev,* Vol. 3, (2002), CD001695, ISSN: 1469-493X

Nasr, A.; Langer, J.C. & Canadian Pediatric Surgery Network. (2011). Influence of location of delivery on outcome in neonates with congenital diaphragmatic hernia. *J Pediatr Surg,* Vol. 46, No. 5, (May 2011), pp. 814–816, ISSN: 0022-3468

Neville, H.L.; Jaksic, T.; Wilson, J.M.; Lally, P.A.; Hardin, W.D. Jr.; Hirschl, R.B.; (2003). Bilateral congenital diaphragmatic hernia. *J Pediatr Surg,* Vol. 38, No. 3, (March 2003), pp. 522–524, ISSN: 0022-3468

Nield, T.A.; Langenbacher, D.; Poulsen, M.K. & Platzker, A.C. (2000). Neurodevelopmental outcome at 3.5 years of age in children treated with extracorporeal life support: relationship to primary diagnosis. *J Pediatr,* Vol. 136, No. 3, (March 2000), pp. 338-344, ISSN: 0022-3476

Ninos, A.; Pierrakakis, S.; Stavrianos, V.; Papaioanou, G.; Ajiazi, A.; Iordanou, C.; Vagenas, P.; Vidali, M.; Douridas, G. & Setakis, N. (2006). Bilateral congenital anterior diaphragmatic hernia: a case report. *Hernia,* Vol. 10, No. 6, (December 2006), pp. 525–527, ISSN: 1265-4906

Nio, M.; Haase, G.; Kennaugh, J.; Bui, K. & Atkinson, J.B. (1994). A prospective randomized trial of delayed versus immediate repair of congenital diaphragmatic hernia. *J Pediatr Surg,* Vol. 29, No. 5, (May, 1994), pp. 618-621, ISSN: 0022-3468

Nishie, A.; Tajima, T.; Asayama, Y.; Ishigami, K.; Hirakawa, M.; Nakayama, T.; Ushijima, Y.; Kakihara, D.; Okamoto, D.; Yoshiura, T.; Masumoto, K.; Taguchi, T.; Tsukimori, K.; Tokunaga, S.; Irie, H.; Yoshimitsu, K. & Honda, H. (2009). MR prediction of postnatal outcomes in left-sided congenital diaphragmatic hernia using right lung signal intensity: comparison with that using right lung volume. *J Magn Reson Imaging,* Vol. 30, No. 1, (July 2009), pp. 112–120, ISSN: 1053-1807

Nobuhara, K.K.; Lund, D.P.; Mitchell, J.; Kharasch, V. & Wilson, J.M. (1996). Long-term outlook for survivors of congenital diaphragmatic hernia. *Clin Perinatol,* Vol. 23, No. 4, (December 1996), pp. 873-887, ISSN: 0095-5108

Norden, M.A.; Butt, W. & McDougall, P. (1994). Predictors of survival for neonates with congenital diaphragmatic hernia. *J Pediatr Surg,* Vol. 29, No. 11, (November 1994), pp. 1442–1446, ISSN: 0022-3468

Okazaki, T.; Okawada, M.; Shiyanagi, S.; Shoji, H.; Shimizu, T.; Tanaka, T.; Takeda, S.; Kawashima, K.; Lane, G.J. & Yamataka, A. (2008). Significance of pulmonary artery size and blood flow as a predictor of outcome in congenital diaphragmatic hernia. *Pediatr Surg Int,* Vol. 24, No. 12, (December 2008), pp. 1369–1373, ISSN: 0179-0358

Ontario Congenital Anomalies Study Group. (2004). Apparent truth about congenital diaphragmatic hernia: a population-based database is needed to establish benchmarking for clinical outcomes for CDH. *J Pediatr Surg,* Vol. 39, No. 5, (May 2004) pp. 661-665, ISSN: 0022-3468

Peetsold, M.G.; Heij, H.A.; Kneepkens, C.M.; Nagelkerke, A.F.; Huisman, J. & Gemke, R.J. (2009). The long-term follow-up of patients with a congenital diaphragmatic hernia: a broad spectrum of morbidity. *Pediatr Surg Int,* Vol. 25, No. 1, (January 2009), pp. 1-17, ISSN: 0179-0358

Peralta, C.F.; Cavoretto, P.; Csapo, B.; Vandecruys, H. & Nicolaides, K.H. (2005). Assessment of lung area in normal fetuses at 12-32 weeks. *Ultrasound Obstet Gynecol,* Vol. 26, No. 7, (December 2005), pp. 718-724, ISSN: 0960-7692

Radhakrishnan, R.S. & Cox, J.C.S. (2005). ECLS and the systemic inflammatory response, In: ECMO: *Extracorporeal cardiopulmonary support in critical care.* (3rd Edition), Van Meurs, K.; Lally, K.P.; Peek, G.J. & Zwischenberger, J.B., editors, pp. 59-83, ELSO, ISBN-10: 0965675629, Ann Arbor, Mitchigan

Reiss, I.; Schaible, T.; van den Hout, L.; Capolupo, I.; Allegaert, K.; van Heijst, A.; Gorett Silva, M.; Greenough, A.; Tibboel, D. & CDH EURO consortium. (2010). Standardized Postnatal Management of Infants with Congenital Diaphragmatic Hernia in Europe: The CDH EURO Consortium Consensus. *Neonatology,* Vol. 98, No. 4, (October 2010), pp. 354–364, ISSN: 1661-7800

Rozmiarek, A.G., Qureshi, F.G.; Cassidy, L.; Ford, H.R. & Hackam, D.J. (2004). Factors Inuencing Survival in Newborns With Congenital Diaphragmatic Hernia: The Relative Role of Timing of Surgery. *J Pediatr Surg,* Vol. 39, No. 6, (June 2004), pp. 821-824, ISSN: 0022-3468

Ruano, R.; de Fatima Yukie Maeda M.; Ikeda Niigaki, J. & Zugaib M. (2007). Pulmonary artery diameters in healthy fetuses from 19–40 weeks gestation. *J Ultrasound Med,* Vol. 26, No. 3, (March 2007), pp. 309–316, ISSN: ISSN: 0278-4297

Saifuddin, A. & Arthur, R. (1993). Congenital diaphragmatic hernia-A review of pre- and postoperative chest radiology. *Clin Radiol,* Vo. 47, No. 2, (February 1993), pp. 104-110, ISSN: 0009-9260

Sakai, H.; Tamura, M.; Hosokawa, Y.; Bryan, A.C.; Barker, G.A. & Bohn, D.J. (1987). Effect of surgical repair on respiratory mechanics in congenital diaphragmatic hernia. *J Pediatr,* Vol. 111, No. 3, (September 1987), pp. 432–438, ISSN: 0022-3476

Sakurai, Y.; Azarow, K.; Cutz, E.; Messineo, A.; Pearl, R. & Bohn, D. (1999). Pulmonary barotrauma in congenital diaphragmatic hernia: a clinicopathological correlation. *J Pediatr Surg,* Vol. 34, No. 12, (December 1999), pp. 1813–1817, ISSN: 0022-3468

Sameroff, A.J. (1998). Environmental risk factors in infancy. *Pediatrics,* Vol. 102, No. 5 Suppl E, (November 1998), pp.1287–1292, ISSN: 0031-4005

Sbragia, L.; Paek, B.W.; Filly, R.A.; Harrison, M.R.; Farrell, J.A.; Farmer, D.L. & Albanese, C.T. (2000). Congenital diaphragmatic hernia without herniation of the liver: does the lung-to-head ratio predict survival? *J Ultrasound Med,* Vol. 19, No. 12, (December 2000), pp. 845-848, ISSN: 0278-4297

Schaible, T.; Kohl, T.; Reinshagen, K.; Brade, J.; Stressig, R. & Büsing, K.A. (2012). Right- versus left-sided congenital diaphragmatic hernia-postnatal outcome at a specialized tertiary care center. *Pediatr Crit Care Med,* Vol. 13, No. 1, (January 2012), pp. 66-71, ISSN: 15297535

Schumacher, R.E.; Palmer, T.W.; Roloff, D.W.; LaClaire, P.A. & Bartlett, R.H. (1991). Follow-up of infants treated with extracorporeal membrane oxygenation for newborn respiratory failure. *Pediatrics,* Vol. 87, No. 4, (April 1991), pp. 451–457, ISSN: 0031-4005

Seetharamaiah, R.; Younger, J.G.; Bartlett, R.H.; Hirschl, R.B. & Congenital Diaphragmatic Hernia Study Group. (2009). Factors associated with survival in infants with congenital diaphragmatic hernia requiring extracorporeal membrane oxygenation: a report from the Congenital Diaphragmatic Hernia Study Group. *J Pediatr Surg,* Vol. 44, No., (July 2009), pp. 1315–1321, ISSN: 0022-3468

Sinha, C.K.; Islam, S.; Patel, S.; Nicolaides, K.; Greenough, A. & Davenport, M. (2009). Congenital diaphragmatic hernia: prognostic indices in the fetal endoluminal tracheal occlusion era. *J Pediatr Surg,* Vol. 44, No. 2, (February 2009), pp. 312-316, ISSN: 0022-3468

Skari, H.; Bjornland, K.; Haugen, G.; Egeland, T. & Emblem, R. (2000). Congenital Diaphragmatic Hernia: A Meta-Analysis of Mortality Factors. *J Pediatr Surg,* Vol. 35, No. 8 (August 2000), pp. 1187-1197, ISSN: 0022-3468

Skari, H.; Bjornland, K.; Frenckner, B.; Friberg, L.G.; Heikkinen, M.; Hurme, T.; Loe, B.; Mollerlokken, G.; Nielsen, O.H.; Qvist, N.; Rintala, R.; Sandgren, K.; Wester, T. & Emblem, R. (2002). Congenital diaphragmatic hernia in Scandinavia from 1995 to 1998: predictors of mortality. *J Pediatr Surg,* Vol. 37, No. 9, (September 2002), pp. 1269-1275, ISSN: 0022-3468

Skari, H.; Bjornland, K.; Frenckner, B.; Friberg, L.G.; Heikkinen, M.; Hurme, T.; Loe, B.; Mollerlokken, G.; Nielsen, O.H.; Qvist, N.; Rintala, R.; Sandgren, K., Serlo, W.; Wagner, K.; Wester, T. & Emblem, R. (2004). Congenital diaphragmatic hernia: a survey of practice in Scandinavia. Pediatr Surg Int, Vol. 20, No. 5, (May 2004), pp. 309–313, ISSN: 0179-0358

Skarsgard, E.D.; MacNab, Y.C.; Qiu, Z.; Little, R.; Lee, S.K. & Canadian Neonatal Network. (2005). SNAP-II predicts mortality among infants with congenital diaphragmatic hernia. *J Perinatol,* Vol. 25, No. 5, (May 2005), pp. 315-319, ISSN: 0743-8346

Sokol, J.; Shimizu, N.; Bohn, D.; Doherty, D.; Ryan, G. & Hornberger, L.K. (2006). Fetal pulmonary artery diameter measurements as a predictor of morbidity in antenatally diagnosed congenital diaphragmatic hernia: a prospective study. *Am J Obstet Gynecol,* Vol. 195, No. 2, (2006), pp. 470–477, ISSN: 0002-9378

Sola, J.E.; Bronson, S.N.; Cheung, M.C.; Ordonez, B.; Neville, H.L. & Koniaris, L.G. (2010). Survival disparities in newborns with congenital diaphragmatic hernia: a national perspective. *J Pediatr Surg,* Vol. 45, No. 6, (June 2010), pp. 1336–1342, ISSN: 0022-3468

Sreenan, C.; Etches, P. & Osiovich, H. (2001). The western Canadian experience with congenital diaphragmatic hernia: perinatal factors predictive of extracorporeal membrane oxygenation and death. *Pediatr Surg Int,* Vol. 17, No. 2-3, (March 2001), pp.196-200, ISSN: 0179-0358

Stege, G.; Fenton, A. & Jaffray, B. (2003). Nihilism in the 1990s: the true mortality of congenital diaphragmatic hernia. *Pediatrics,* Vol. 112, No. 3 Pt 1, (September 2003), pp. 532–535, ISSN: 0031-4005

Stevens, T.P.; Chess, P.R.; McConnochie, K.M.; Sinkin, R.A.; Guillet, R.; Maniscalco, W.M. & Fisher, S.G. (2002). Survival in early- and late-term infants with congenital diaphragmatic hernia treated with extracorporeal membrane oxygenation. *Pediatrics,* Vol. 110, No. 3, (September 2002); pp. 590- 596, ISSN: 0031-4005

Stevens, T.P.; van Wijngaarden, E.; Ackerman, K.G.; Lally, P.A.; Lally, K.P. & Congenital Diaphragmatic Hernia Study Group. (2009). Timing of delivery and survival rates for infants with prenatal diagnoses of congenital diaphragmatic hernia. *Pediatrics,* Vol. 123, No. 2, (February 2009), pp. 494-502, ISSN: 0031-4005

Stolar, C.J.; Crisa, M.A. & Driscoll, Y.T. (1995). Neurocognitive outcome for neonates treated with extracorporeal membrane oxygenation: are infants with congenital diaphragmatic hernia different? *J Pediatr Surg,* Vol. 30, No. 2, (February 1995), pp. 366-371, ISSN: 0022-3468

Suda, K., Bigras, J.L., Bohn, D., Hornberger, L.K. & McCrindle, B.W. (2000). Echocardiographic predictors of outcome in newborns with congenital diaphragmatic hernia. *Pediatrics,* Vol. 105, No. 5, (May 2000), pp. 1106-1109, ISSN: 0031-4005

Terui, K.; Omoto, A.; Osada, H.; Hishiki, T.; Saito, T.; Sato, Y.; Nakata, M.; Komatsu, S.; Ono, S. & Yoshida, H. (2011). Prediction of postnatal outcomes in congenital diaphragmatic hernia using MRI signal intensity of the fetal lung. *J Perinatol,* Vol. 31, No. 4, (April 2011), pp. 269–273, ISSN: 0743-8346

Tiruvoipati, R.; Vinogradova, Y.; Faulkner, G.; Sosnowski, A.W.; Firmin, R.K. & Peek, G.J. (2007). Predictors of outcome in patients with congenital diaphragmatic hernia requiring extracorporeal membrane oxygenation. *J Pediatr Surg,* Vol. 42, No.8, (August 2007), pp. 1345-1350, ISSN: 0022-3468

Touloukian, R.J. & Markowitz, R. (1984). A preoperative x-ray scoring system for risk assessment of newborns with congenital diaphragmatic hernia. *J Pediatr Surg,* Vol. 19, No. 3, (June 1984), pp. 252–257, ISSN: 0022-3468

Towne, B.H.; Lott, I.T.; Hicks, D.A. & Healey, T. (1985). Long-term follow-up of infants and children treated with extracorporeal membrane oxygenation (ECMO): a preliminary report. *J Pediatr Surg,* Vol. 20, No. 4, (August 1985), pp. 410–414, ISSN: 0022-3468

Tsao, K.J.; Allison, N.D.; Harting, M.T.; Lally, P.A. & Lally, K.P. (2010). Congenital diaphragmatic hernia in the preterm infant. *Surgery,* Vol. 148, No. 2, (August 2010), pp. 404-410, ISSN: 0263-9319

Usui, N.; Okuyama, H.; Sawai, T.; Kamiyama, M.; Kamata, S. & Fukuzawa, M. (2007). Relationship between L/T ratio and LHR in the prenatal assessment of pulmonary hypoplasia in congenital diaphragmatic hernia. *Pediatr Surg Int,* Vol. 23, No. 10, (October 2007); pp. 971–976, ISSN: 0179-0358

Valfrè, L.; Braguglia, A.; Conforti, A.; Morini, F.; Trucchi, A.; Iacobelli, B.D.; Nahom, A.; Chukhlantseva, N.; Dotta, A.; Corchia, C. & Bagolan, P. (2011). Long term follow-up in high-risk congenital diaphragmatic hernia survivors: patching the diaphragm affects the outcome. *J Pediatr Surg,* Vol. 45, No. 1, (January 2011), pp. 52-56, ISSN: 0022-3468

Wilson, J.M.; Lund, D.P.; Lillehei, C.W.; & Vacanti JP. (1997). Congenital diaphragmatic hernia A tale of two cities: The Boston experience. *J Pediatr Surg,* Vol. 32, No. 3, (March 1997), pp. 401-405, ISSN: 0022-3468

Wright, J.E.; Budd, J.L.S.; Field, D.J. & Draper, E.S. (2010). Epidemiology and outcome of congenital diaphragmatic hernia: a 9-year experience. *Paediatr Perinat Epidemiol,* Vol. 25, No. 2, (March 2010), pp. 144–149, ISSN: 1365-3016

Wung, J.T.; James, L.S.; Kilchevsky, E. & James E. (1985). Management of infants with severe respiratory failure and persistence of the fetal circulation, without hyperventilation. *Pediatrics,* Vol. 76, No. 4, (October, 1985), pp. 488-494, ISSN: 0031-4005

Wung, J.T.; Sahni, R.; Moffitt, S.T.; Lipsitz, E. & Stolar, C.J. (1995). Congenital diaphragmatic hernia: survival treated with very delayed surgery, spontaneous respiration, and no chest tube. *J Pediatr Surg,* Vol. 30, No. 3, (March 1995), pp. 406-409, ISSN: 0022-3468

Yang, S.H.; Nobuhara, K.K.; Keller, R.L.; Ball, R.H.; Goldstein, R.B.; Feldstein, V.A.; Callen, P.W.; Filly, R.A.; Farmer, D.L.; Harrison, M.R. & Lee, H. (2007). Reliability of the lung-to-head ratio as a predictor of outcome in fetuses with isolated left congenital diaphragmatic hernia at gestation outside 24-26 weeks. *Am J Obstet Gynecol,* Vol. 197, No. 1, (July 2007), pp. 30.e1-7, ISSN: 0002-9378

Yang, W.; Carmichael, S.L.; Harris, J.A. & Shaw, G.M. (2006). Epidemiologic characteristics of congenital diaphragmatic hernia among 2.5 million California births, 1989–1997. *Birth Defects Res A Clin Mol Teratol,* Vol. 76, No. 3, (March 2006); pp. 170–174, ISSN: 1542- 0752, 1542-0760

Zaiss, I.; Kehl, S.; Link, K.; Neff, W.; Schaible, T.; Sütterlin, M.; Siemer, J. (2011). Associated Malformations in Congenital Diaphragmatic Hernia. *Am J Perinatol,* Vol. 28, No. 3, (March 2011), pp. 211-218, ISSN: 0743-8346